Mayada Jemaa
Yomn Ben Hmidene

The power of the Erbium laser in conservative dentistry and endodontics

Mayada Jemaa
Yomn Ben Hmidene

The power of the Erbium laser in conservative dentistry and endodontics

Imprint

Any brand names and product names mentioned in this book are subject to trademark, brand or patent protection and are trademarks or registered trademarks of their respective holders. The use of brand names, product names, common names, trade names, product descriptions etc. even without a particular marking in this work is in no way to be construed to mean that such names may be regarded as unrestricted in respect of trademark and brand protection legislation and could thus be used by anyone.

Cover image: www.ingimage.com

This book is a translation from the original published under ISBN 978-620-6-71340-1.

Publisher:
Sciencia Scripts
is a trademark of
Dodo Books Indian Ocean Ltd. and OmniScriptum S.R.L publishing group

120 High Road, East Finchley, London, N2 9ED, United Kingdom
Str. Armeneasca 28/1, office 1, Chisinau MD-2012, Republic of Moldova, Europe
Printed at: see last page
ISBN: 978-620-7-62620-5

Table of contents

Introduction

Introduction

Since their first appearance in 1960, LASER systems have gone from strength to strength, and are now one of the most widely used technologies.

Used in a wide range of fields, LASER has well and truly carved out a place for itself in the healthcare sector as a diagnostic and therapeutic tool [23].

The first medical LASER was a Ruby LASER. Later, with the introduction of different types of LASER, its indications were gradually extended to several medical specialties, including modern dentistry.

Indeed, the first use of lasers for dental cavity preparation was described in 1964 with the Ruby laser (693.4 nm). In the following years, other lasers with different wavelengths were evaluated, such as Nd:YAG (1.065 μm) and CO_2 (9.6 μm). The major disadvantages of the latter are firstly their low absorption in dental tissue, thus reducing their effectiveness, but also an increase in temperature within the pulp causing tissue carbonization and the appearance of microcracks [23,86].

In recent decades, the appearance on the market of the Erbium family of lasers, with their two wavelengths of 2940 nm and 2780 nm, has enabled professionals in the field to overcome these drawbacks. Indeed, thanks to their strong absorption in water and hydroxyapatite, Erbium : Yttrium Aluminium Garnet (Er: YAG) and Erbium, Chromium : Yttrium, Scandium, Gallium, Garnet (Er, Cr: YSGG) lasers, since the first work by Keller and Hibst in 1989, have proven their effectiveness on both hard and soft tooth tissues [13,82].

In addition, thanks to their versatility, these lasers have been extensively studied, and are currently the lasers of choice for various conservative tooth treatments, such as caries curettage, preparation of bonding cavities and treatment of dentine hypersensitivity.

In endodontics, Erbium lasers are also increasingly indicated in the various phases of root canal treatment. On the one hand, they overcome the difficulties encountered during conventional endodontic treatment (anatomical complexities and the inability of irrigation solutions to penetrate lateral canals and apical ramifications) and, on the other, they offer the possibility of enhancing the capacity to clean and eliminate root canal debris, thus ensuring better decontamination of the endodontic system [64].

The main aim of our work was therefore to evaluate the contribution of each of the two Erbium lasers (Er: YAG and Er, Cr: YSGG) in Conservative Odontology and Endodontics (COE), in an attempt to conclude, based on recent data in the literature, which of these two lasers is best suited to this specialty.

In order to meet this objective, the first chapter presents the two Er:YAG and Er,Cr:YSGG lasers, their main characteristics and their various clinical applications. The second chapter describes the effects of these two Erbium lasers on dental tissue. This was followed by two main chapters detailing the contribution of Er: YAG and Er, Cr: YSGG lasers to conservative dentistry and endodontics. In the final chapter, we compare these two lasers and conclude, with reference to the data in the literature, which of the two is the most useful in our OCE practice.

Erbium lasers (Er: YAG and Er, Cr: YSGG)

1. Introducing Erbium lasers [1,23,93].

The erbium laser family, which includes lasers with a solid active medium (crystal), is essentially represented by 3 types of lasers emitting in the mid-infrared:

- *Er: YAG laser* (Erbium: Yttrium-Aluminium-Garnet) with a wavelength of 2.49 µm.

- *Er, Cr: YSGG laser* (Erbium, Chromium: Yttrium-ScandiumGadolinium-Garnet) with a wavelength of 2.78µm.

- *Er laser: YSGG* (Erbium: Yttrium-Scandium-Gadolinium-Garnet) with a wavelength of 2.79µm.

The *garnets* found in the composition of the laser's amplifying medium are crystalline solids.

2. Advantages and disadvantages (Table N°I)

Table I: Advantages and disadvantages of Erbium lasers in dental practice [1,70,71,85].

Benefits	Disadvantages

-Indicated for the treatment of hard and soft dental tissue. -Minimally invasive therapy (ablation) selective fabrics). -Little or no local anaesthetic required. -No noise or vibration during processing. -Efficient sludge removal Smear Layer. -Surface decontamination. -Little heating of pulp tissue. -Less risk of iatrogenic damage.	-Slower processing time than conventional techniques. -Weak hemostatic action in surgery. - Requires intensive training in operation and settings. -Their use is dangerous if the necessary precautions are not taken. -High cost.

3. The Er: YAG laser

3.1. Definition [1,13,16,93]

The Er: YAG laser uses a solid active medium of yttrium-aluminum garnet (Y3Al5O12) doped with ions (Er3+) that are only Lanthanides (a group of rare earths). It operates via an optical pumping system characterized by an intense flash of light corresponding to an absorption band of the Er3+ ion incorporated in the crystal.
This laser emits in the mid-infrared at a wavelength of 2940 nm, which corresponds to the absorption peak of both water and hydroxyapatite. The result is excellent absorption by enamel, dentin and soft tissue. One of the main features of the Er:YAG laser is its low tissue penetration and controlled thermal effect.

❖ *An example of an Er: YAG laser*: Syneron's LiteTouch™ laser

(Figure 1).

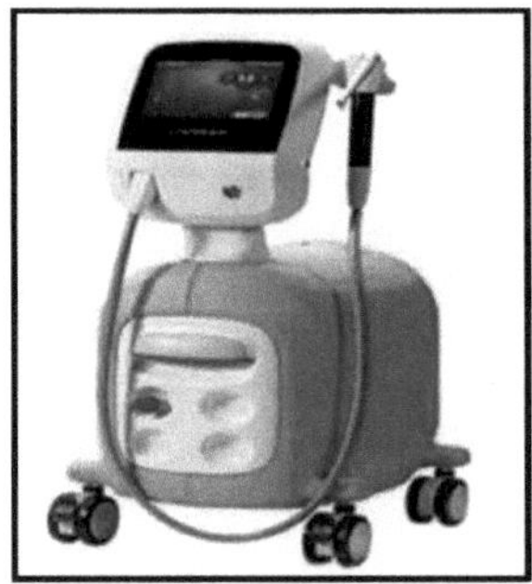

Figure 1: The Er: YAG LiteTouch™ laser (Syneron) [1].

3.2 Characteristics [2,13,68].

Active medium	Yttrium-aluminum garnet doped with ErbiumEr3+ ions
Wavelength	2940 nm
Transmission mode	Pulsed
Pulse duration	50µs to 1000µs
Transmission mode	Sapphire- or quartz-based flexible optical fiber -Articulated arm

In 2005, Bertrand and Rocca compared the light transmission efficiency of the Er:YAG laser using fiber optics and the articulated mirror arm. They found that the latter required working at a distance from the target tissue, with a focal distance to be respected of the order of 9 to 15 mm. Below or above this distance, there was a risk of losing some of the ablation potential.

What's more, the authors revealed that the mirrors clog up very quickly and need to be cleaned regularly with a compress.

On the other hand, it has been reported that the use of a quartz or sapphire tip offers the advantage of being able to work in contact with dental tissues without the need for a focal length [13].

3.3. Clinical applications [2,93]

Table II: Clinical applications of Er:YAG and Er,Cr:YSGG lasers.

Dentistry Curator	- Caries removal - Preparing bonding cavities - Enamel and dentin conditioning - Well and crack sealing - Desensitization of sensitive dental necks
Endodontics	- Root canal preparation and cleaning - Activation of endodontic irrigation solutions - Endodontic surgery (apical resection)
Periodontology	- Sulcular debridement - Periodontal pocket decontamination - Coronary elongation - Drilling in implantology (not precise enough)
Oral surgery	- Soft-tissue surgery (incision, excision, coagulation) - Freinectomy - Deepening the vestibules - Elimination of pathological tissue (cysts, neoplasms, etc.) and hyperplastic tissue (granulation tissue) around the apex - Treatment of ulcers - Osteotomy, osteoplasty

4. Er, Cr laser: YSGG

4.1. Definition [1,16]

The Er, Cr: YSGG laser also emits in the mid-infrared at a wavelength of 2,780 nm. Its active medium is an yttrium scandium galium garnet crystal doped with Erbium (Er3+) ions.

It has almost the same properties as the Er: YAG laser, except that its wavelength is slightly less absorbed by water but more absorbed by hydroxyl ions (Figure 2).

This makes its penetration of dental tissue 3 times greater than that of the Er:YAG laser.

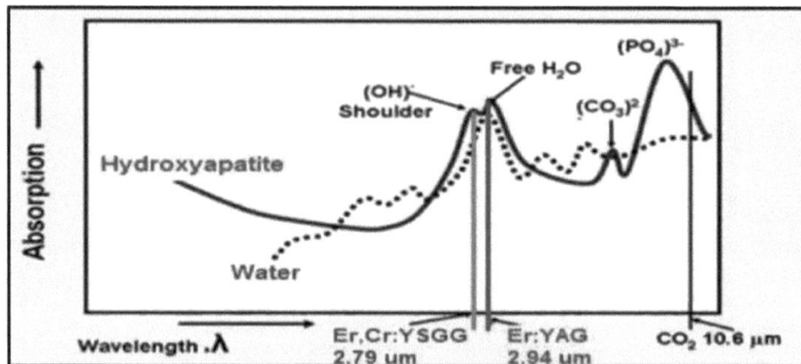

Figure 2: Absorption of Erbium wavelengths in hard dental tissue chromophores [1].

❖ *Example of an Er, Cr: YSGG laser:* Biolase's WaterlaseiPlus® laser.

(USA). (Figure 3)

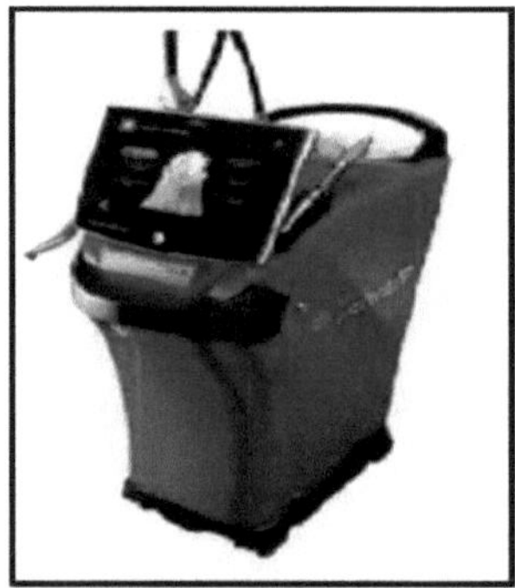

Figure 3: The Er, Cr: YSGG WaterlaseiPlus® laser from Biolase [1].

4.2. Features [2,68]

Active medium	Yttrium scandium gallium garnet crystal doped with erbium chromium

Wavelength	2780 nm
Transmission mode	Pulsed
Pulse duration	>500µs
Transmission mode	Optical fiber

4.3. Clinical applications

The clinical applications of the Er, Cr: YSGG laser are identical to those of the Er: YAG laser, previously detailed in Table II.

Effects of Erbium lasers on dental tissue

1. Effects on enamel

In 2010, Tsanova and Tomov studied the morphological changes in tooth enamel irradiated with the Er:YAG laser using a Scanning Electron Microscope (SEM). They found that, following irradiation, the enamel showed a typical appearance of a rough, irregular surface similar to that etched with acid, with enamel prisms grouped in so-called *"honeycomb"* clusters [87].

Similarly, Darlon Martins et al in 2014 revealed following Scanning Electron Microscope (SEM) studies performed on human enamel irradiated with an Er: YAG laser, rough surfaces with enamel prisms ejected by laser ablation effect [51].

Indeed, these authors reported that, due to the high absorption rate of Erbium beams by water in the interprismal space, exposure of enamel prisms was produced after irradiation (Figure 4).

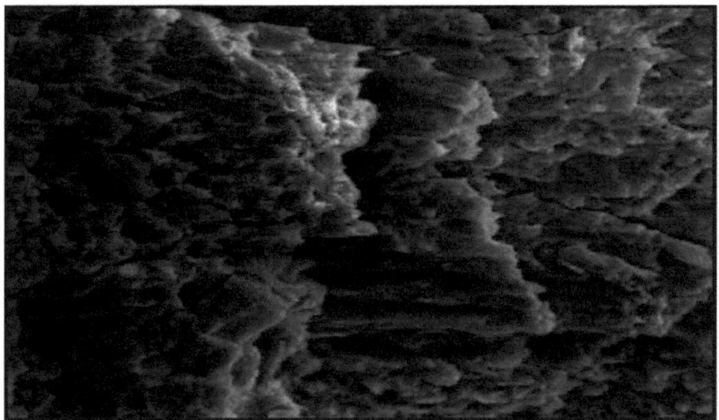

**Figure 4: SEM view of enamel exposed to Er: YAG laser (magnification ×
1000) [51].**

With the Er, Cr: YSGG laser, Mozammal et al in 2001 found that irradiated enamel also had a rough surface, with prominent "*ladder*" enamel prisms and no signs of erosion or fusion [35] (Figure 5).

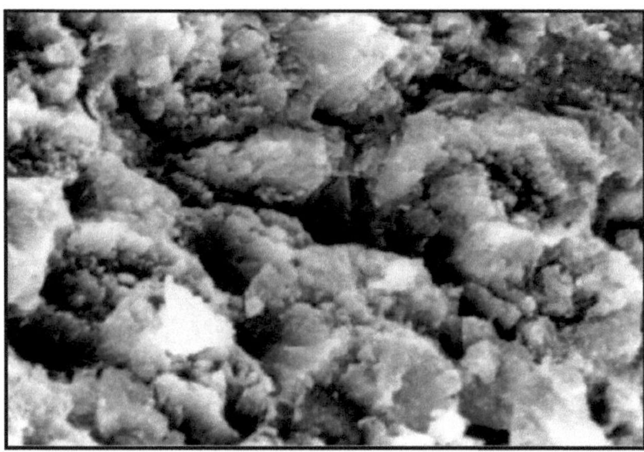

Figure 5: SEM view of enamel exposed to Er, Cr: YSGG laser (magnification × 5000) [35].

The study by Harashima et al in 2005 revealed that the two lasers Er: YAG (2940nm) and Er, Cr: YSGG (2780nm), given their very close wavelengths, show almost similar morphological results in enamel irradiated and observed by SEM [34].

However, it was reported in the same study that tooth surfaces irradiated with the Er, Cr: YSGG laser were rougher than those irradiated with the Er: YAG laser.

This difference in roughness was justified by the fact that surfaces irradiated by the Er, Cr: YSGG laser were more thermally affected than those irradiated by the Er: YAG laser (enamel ablation was initiated at temperatures of around 800°C for the Er, Cr: YSGG and300°C for the Er: YAG) [34].

2. Effects on dentine

Studies by Tomomi Hrashima et al in 2005,Shi et al in 2009, Shi Lin et al in 2010 and Darlon Martins et al in 2014, demonstrated that Erbium laser irradiation was more effective in dentin tissue than at the enamel level, due to the presence of a large amount of water in dentin [34,51,52].

Indeed, according to Shi Lin et al in 2010, dentin, which is composed of 20% water by volume, absorbs more Erbium wavelengths than dental enamel (containing no more than 12% water by volume). As a result, the ablation rate of dentin was faster than that of dental enamel, and the power parameters used were lower [52].

Darlon Martins et al in 2014, evaluated the effect of the Er: YAG laser (2940nm) on dentin surface morphology. Following SEM analysis, they noted the alteration of dentin microstructure with an irregular surface appearance, devoid of dentin sludge with widely open dentin tubules and prominent peritubular dentin (Figure 6).

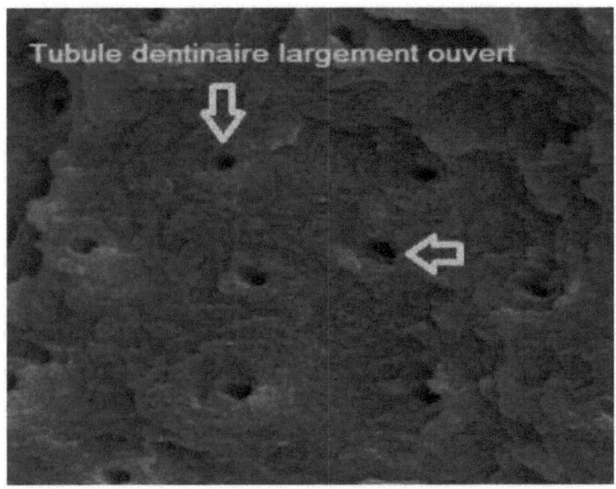

The authors also revealed that intertubular dentin, due to its water-rich content, underwent greater ablation than peritubular dentin, hence the prominent appearance of dentinal tubules [51].

Previous studies, such as those by Matsumoto et al in 2003, Ramos et al in 2004 and Corona et al in 2007, have suggested that the dentin surface appearance obtained by irradiation with Erbium lasers would be favorable for dentin bonding procedures compared to other types of lasers.

In fact, it was mentioned in these studies that the absence of a smear layer and wide-open dentinal tubules could potentially increase dentin permeability and therefore favour the infiltration of resin monomers into the dentin tissue.

Nevertheless, more recent studies have shown that the effect of irradiation on the dentin surface, prior to the bonding procedure, can reveal divergent results depending on the laser parameters used [12,52].

3. Effects on the pulp

Undesirable thermal effects on pulp tissue are probably the biggest problem when treating hard dental tissue.

However, as far back as the earlier studies by Keller and Hibst in 1998, it was proven that dental tissue could be removed with the Er: YAG laser without causing any thermal damage to the pulp, provided that the appropriate laser parameters were used and a suitable water spray was employed.

In addition, studies by Takamori et al. in 2000 and Martins et al. in 2005 reported that an increase in pulp temperature could be observed after Er: YAG laser irradiation, but not exceeding 5.5°C (critical pulp temperature at which pulp vitality will be compromised).

The study by Kilini et al in 2009, whose aim was to compare the thermal safety of the two Er: YAG and Er, Cr: YSGG lasers with that of diamond burs, showed that Erbium lasers, although generating significantly less heat at the irradiated tooth surfaces compared with burs, both lasers produce a greater increase in temperature at pulpal level [42].

However, this temperature rise always remains below the critical value (5.5°C) for both systems, and does not cause thermal damage to the dental pulp [42].

Also, Raucci-Neto et al in 2014, showed that the increase in temperature during ablation of healthy and demineralized dental tissue correlated with the energy level employed from the Er: YAG laser. Thus, groups of teeth irradiated with energies of 200 and 250 mJ revealed the highest temperature values (between 3.5 and4.5°C) [73].

Nevertheless, none of the energy parameters used resulted in a temperature increase in excess of 5°C. Consequently, the authors were able to conclude that the use of the Erbium laser for hard tissue ablation cannot be considered as a potential source of thermal damage to the pulp.

Erbium lasers (Er: YAÇ and Er, Cr: YSÇÇ) in conservative dentistry

1. Prevention of Erbium laser-induced demineralization "LIPD

The possibility of increasing the acid resistance of enamel after laser irradiation, commonly referred to as *"Laser Induced Prevention of Demineralization"* (LIPD), was first described in 1965 with the ruby laser [72].

Consequently, several authors have reported on the effect of preventing tooth demineralization with different wavelengths chosen according to their absorption in hard dental tissue (Castellan et al. 2007; De Freitas et al. 2010; Correa-Afonso et al. 2012).

Given the volume composition of dental enamel: 85% hydroxyapatite, 12% water and 3% proteins and lipids, the use of wavelengths strongly absorbed by water and hydroxyapatite was capable of generating thermal changes in enamel, resulting in a chemical modification of its structure and an increase in its resistance to acid attack [31,72].

Similarly, for dentin, laser irradiation strongly absorbed by the chromophores of this tissue (especially water) was likely to improve resistance to acid attack and inhibit the progression of caries at the dentinal level [72].

For example, Er:YAG and Er,Cr:YSGG lasers, which operate at the wavelengths most absorbed by hard dental tissue, have been extensively studied in the context of preventing dental demineralization.

► **Mechanism of action**

To date, the exact mechanism by which Er: YAG (2.94μm) and Er,

Cr: YSGG (2.78μm) lasers act on the tooth surface, increasing its resistance to demineralization, is not well established in the literature. Nevertheless, authors have suggested that two main mechanisms are responsible for the reduced solubility of tooth enamel irradiated with Erbium lasers [72].

The first mechanism, according to the authors, concerns changes in the chemical composition of dental enamel, which occur when the temperature at the enamel surface, irradiated with Erbium lasers, rises from 100 to 650°C, leading to a reduction in water and carbonate content on the one hand, and an increase in hydroxyl ions and the formation of pyrophosphates on the other (Geraldo-Martin, 2013; Diaz-Monroy et al. 2014 ;Colucci et al. 2015).

Diaz-Monroy et al (2014) conducted an in vitro study with the aim of assessing changes in the structure of tooth enamel irradiated with Er: YAG laser.

They concluded that enamel resistance to acid dissolution was mainly associated with a change in its mineral composition, namely a significant reduction in the percentage of carbon (C) and an increase in oxygen (O), phosphorus (P) and calcium (Ca). [29]

These same changes were observed by Ceballos-Jiménez et al. in 2018, who showed that Er: YAG laser irradiation alone or combined with fluoride gel application could promote the acid resistance of tooth enamel by increasing the Ca/P ratio, considered the most reliable indicator of tooth demineralization [18].

On the other hand, Muller Ramalho et al. in 2015 reported that the carbonate ion, present in the mineral composition of enamel, integrates poorly into the network of hydroxyapatite crystals and gives rise to an apatite phase that is less stable and therefore more soluble in acids. Irradiation with Erbium lasers therefore had the role of eliminating, by photothermal effect, this mineral substance considered an impurity, thus reducing the degree of dissolution of dental enamel [72].

With regard to the second mechanism, some authors have shown that during laser irradiation, the partial decomposition of the organic matrix occupying the inter- and intra-prismatic spaces of tooth enamel leads to blockage of the latter. As a result, acid influx and mineral diffusion out of the enamel can be compromised (Ying et al. 2004; Maung et al. 2007; Liu et al. 2012).

Other published studies have supported this "organic blockage" theory [31,62].

Furthermore, a review of the literature has shown that organic matrix fusion induced by irradiation of enamel surfaces with Erbium lasers contributes at least 25% to the inhibition of mineral loss and 57% to the arrest of progression of incipient carious lesions [72].

However, it has been reported that the effect of organic blocking can peak and decrease after complete decomposition of the organic matrix at temperatures >400°C (Geraldo-Martins et al. 2012).

Thus, the efficacy and safety of both Er: YAG (2.94µm) and Er, Cr: YSGG (2.78µm) lasers in preventing dental demineralization was directly related to the proper setting of laser parameters and laser working conditions.

► **Influence of laser parameters in LIPD**

According to the literature review, the optimal energy values for LIPD using Erbium wavelengths have given rise to controversy [72]. An in vitro study by Liu et al. in 2013, conducted to evaluate the cariostatic potential of the Er: YAG laser (2940nm) used at low energy densities, showed that Er: YAG laser irradiation of dental surfaces with sub-ablative energy densities of 2 J/cm^2 and 5.1 J/cm^2 was able to significantly prevent enamel demineralization by 38% compared to the control (non-irradiated) surface without eliminating tissue and without any thermal damage generated.

Nevertheless, the authors reported that treatment at 5.1 J/cm2 was more effective in preventing demineralization (45.2%) than that at 2 J/cm2 (25.2%) [54].

Gerardo-Martins et al in 2013, showed that Er, Cr: YSGG laser irradiation was able to increase the acid resistance of irradiated enamel by 23% compared to the control surface, while using the lowest output power 0.25 W (62.5 J $/cm^2$) and without water and air spraying [31].

For their part, De Oliveira et al in 2017 suggested that a pulse frequency of 30 Hz and an output power of 0.5 W from the Er, Cr: YSGG laser could be considered the best parameters for LIPD [24].

With regard to the contribution of water spray when irradiating dental surfaces with Erbium lasers, satisfactory results in preventing demineralization have been obtained with or without cooling [72].

Indeed, among the studies that have shown positive LIPD results by irradiation with Erbium lasers, some have used water cooling (Correa-Afonso et al in 2010; Colucci et al in 2015) and others have not (Liu et al in 2013).

However, it has been reported that the presence of large quantities of water during laser irradiation increases the risk of ablation, as well as the porosity of the tooth surface, facilitating the diffusion of acids into the enamel structure and increasing the depth of demineralization (Colucci et al in 2009 and Olivi et al in 2010).

Thus, some authors such as Scatolin et al in 2014 and Colucci et al in 2015 have advocated minimum water quantities of 2 to 5ml/min to cool dental surfaces irradiated with Erbium lasers in LIPD.

▶ **Combined treatment: Erbium lasers and remineralization gels**

Several authors have reported the benefit of irradiating dental surfaces with Erbium lasers combined with the application of fluoride-based gels in preventing demineralization of dental tissues (Ana et al. 2012; Liu et al. 2013; Mathew et al .2013).

In 2013, an in vitro study was carried out by Liu et al. with the aim of comparing the cariostatic effect of combined laser-fluoride treatment with laser treatments alone and fluoride treatments alone [53].

The result of this study was in favor of a significant cariostatic effect of the combined treatment compared to other treatments. Low-energy Er:YAG laser irradiation (5.1 J/cm^2) coupled with 2% NaF fluoride gel treatment prevented 54.8% of tooth enamel demineralization, while laser irradiation alone prevented 41.2%, and fluoride alone prevented only 28.9%.

The authors suggested that Er:YAG laser irradiation of tooth surfaces after fluoride treatment could instantly transform enamel thydroxyapatite into fluorinated hydroxyapatite, thereby increasing enamel's resistance to acids [53].

In an in vitro study in 2016, Kumar et al. compared enamel surface strength after Er, Cr: YSGG laser irradiation alone or in combination with fluoride treatment [46].

The Er, Cr : YSGG laser was used with sub-ablative parameters: 2.8 J/cm2 ; 0.5 W ; 20 Hz.

Two types of fluoride gel were used in two different ways: after laser irradiation and as a pretreatment (before irradiation).

- 2% NaF" *Sodium Fluoride* gel
- APF 1.23% *Acidulated Posphate Fluoride* gel

The study showed that :

- There was a marked change in enamel surface topography after laser irradiation: the surface appeared more eroded with craters and fissures, and the synergistic application of the gel resulted in the formation of globules and granules as well as a vitrified appearance of the enamel surface.
- The microhardness value increased more significantly after using the NaF gel than after the APF gel.
- A maximum increase in enamel microhardness was observed when fluoride gel (APF) was applied prior to laser irradiation (as a pretreatment).

The authors concluded that Er, Cr: YSGG laser irradiation alone or in combination with fluoride gel could be an effective tool for increasing enamel resistance to caries [46].

However, the study by Molaasadollah et al in 2017 carried out to compare the efficacy of fluoride gel (APF 1.23%) alone and in combination with the Er, Cr: YSGG laser (0.5 W; 20 Hz) in remineralizing white lesions (white spot) in primary teeth, showed that Er, Cr: YSGG laser irradiation did not enhance the efficacy of fluoride in controlling the progression of these lesions [61].

Indeed, the authors reported that there was no significant difference between the groups of teeth treated with fluoride alone and those in combination with the Er, Cr: YSGG laser in terms of lesion extent.

Thus, although there is much controversial information in the literature regarding the potential of the Erbium laser alone or in combination with other interventions in the prevention of dental demineralization, most publications have reported favorable results [72].

However, information on the optimum energy range used and the protocol to be followed for preventing demineralization using Erbium wavelengths is still required.

2. Caries removal and cavity preparation

Since their use for the treatment of hard dental tissue was approved by the Food and Drug Administration(FDA) in 1997 and 1998 respectively, Er: YAG (2940 nm) and Er, Cr: YSGG (2780 nm) lasers have been widely studied for the removal of decayed tissue and cavity preparation [79].

Antonis Kallis et al. in 2016, reported that the Er: YAG laser was considered the laser of choice for cutting hard dental tissue quickly, efficiently and safely.

Riccardo Poli et al. in 2017, reported that Er: YAG (2940nm) and Er, Cr: YSGG (2780nm) lasers could be used as an alternative to the burr for the removal of carious lesions and the preparation of class I, II, III, IV and V cavities (Black's classification) with the advantage of jointly removing soft tissue, if necessary [71].

An in vitro study by Al-Batayneh et al in 2014 , comparing the cutting efficiency of the Er: YAG laser (2940 nm) versus diamond burs on primary and permanent teeth, showed that higher enamel and dentin ablation rates and significantly more effective removal of decayed tooth tissue were observed after Erbium laser irradiation compared to conventional treatment [10].

This study reported that temperature increases in the pulp did not exceed the threshold of 5.5°C in any tooth during laser ablation. Furthermore, Tao et al in 2017, in a meta-analysis of the literature, revealed that the Erbium laser, in addition to its safety, it reduces the use of local anesthesia during excision of carious tissue compared with conventional burr treatment [85].

Indeed, it has been noted that in most clinical studies, few people in the Er:YAG laser group experienced pain and requested local anaesthesia during cavity preparation.

Furthermore, a clinical study by Zhegova et al in 2015 ,conducted with the aim of evaluating the efficacy of the Er: YAG laser in the treatment of carious lesions in permanent teeth in children aged 6 to 16, showed that after 2 years of follow-up, no postoperative sensitivity or secondary caries were detected in all patients [92].

Also, the study reported that 94.83% of restorations of carious lesions, treated with the Er: YAG laser, were clinically acceptable, and none of the restorations were lost after 2 years.

Er:YAG laser treatment was also more accepted by patients than conventional treatment due to the absence of noise, vibration and the need for anesthesia before and during treatment [92].

2.1. Mechanism of action

The ablation of hard dental tissue by Erbium lasers is the result of a complex mechanism involving two main effects: thermal and mechanical [1].

Indeed, the interaction of Erbium radiation with mineralized dental tissues, whether healthy or decayed, leads to a rise in temperature at the level of the water molecules contained in enamel and dentin.

This results in volumetric expansion and high internal pressure, leading to the elimination of material by micro-explosions [1,13].

This thermomechanical ablation process occurs at temperatures below the melting point of hard dental tissue (1200°C) and varies according to the wavelength of the laser used: the Er: YAG laser (2940 nm) reaches 300°C at the ablation threshold, while the Er, Cr: YSGG laser reaches 800°C (Ana et al. ,2007 ; Neves et al. ,2010).

2.2. Influence of laser parameters on ablation efficiency

According to the literature review, the average threshold level at which ablation of hard dental tissue occurs is around 8 to 11 J/cm^2 for the Er: YAG laser and 10 to 14 J/cm^2 for the Er, Cr: YSGG laser [71]. However, authors such as Laria et al. in 2011 and Strakas et al. in 2018 have shown that the cutting efficiency of Er: YAG and Er, Cr:

YSGG lasers correlates with various parameters such as laser energy, output power and number of pulses per second.

Riccardo Poli et al. in 2017, mentioned that laser energy must be adjusted according to the target tissue involved [71].

The table below (Table III) summarizes the average energies recommended by the author for effective and safe ablation of hard dental tissue by Erbium lasers.

Table III: Erbium laser energy values as a function of target tissue [71].

Fabric	Temporary tooth		Permanent tooth		Dentin Cariée
	Email	Dentin	Email	Dentin	
Energy	100-200 mJ	100-150 mJ	200-250 mJ	100-200 mJ	100-150 mJ

The more water the tissue contains, the less energy it requires to be eliminated. Pulse duration is also a very important parameter to take into account when setting up the laser. The shorter the pulse duration, the lower the energy converted into heat, and the less interaction and thermal damage to dental tissue [71].

An in vitro study by Baraba et al. in 2013, evaluating the ablation rate of the Er: YAG laser in dentin using three different pulse durations, showed that the "clinical ablation rate" measured in mm^i /s, was greater when the Er: YAG laser was used with the SSP "Super Short Pulse" mode (pulses of 50 µs) than with the MSP "Medium Short Pulse" mode (pulses of 100 µs) or the SP "Short Pulse" mode (pulses of 300 µs) [11].

The authors explained these results by the fact that, in SSP mode, the heat had no time to diffuse into the tissue or dissipate, and most of the energy was absorbed by the water and used to ablate the dentin tissue [11].

Adjustment of the pulse repetition rate, also known as pulse frequency (expressed in Hz or pulses per second), is also very important to avoid excessive heating of hard dental tissue.

As the number of pulses per unit of time increases, the interval between pulses (thermal relaxation time) is reduced, leaving less time for cooling dental tissue [1].

Thus, water and air spraying are always necessary during treatment to reduce the temperature of the irradiated site and evacuate the debris removed.

2.3. Ablation selectivity

Minimally invasive cavity preparation relies on the removal of demineralized tissue without sacrificing healthy or potentially remineralizable tissue. (Toro et al. , 2013)

As carious tissues are softer and contain more water than healthy dental tissues, their removal by Erbium wavelengths (2490 nm and 2780nm) was easier, more conservative and with minimal heat transfer compared to underlying healthy tissues [71].

Matos et al. in 2012, reported that Er: YAG and Er, Cr: YSGG lasers, due to their high affinity with water, selectively remove demineralized dental tissue without extending the preparation into healthy structures [56].

Riccardo Poli et al in 2017, reported that the Erbium laser used in the treatment of carious lesions enables efficient and rapid removal of carious tissue while preserving healthy tissue [71].

Nevertheless, authors such as Eberhard et al. in 2008; Tao et al. in 2009 have reported that it is often difficult for the practitioner to determine the end point of demineralized tissue ablation by Erbium lasers.

In some cases, this may require the use of laser fluorescence diagnostic equipment for selective removal of infected dentine [56,82].

This is a diode laser which emits at a wavelength of 655 nm (red light). The principle behind this application is that the fluorescence of healthy tissue differs from that of carious tissue due to variations in its chemical composition, such as the presence of proteins, bacteria and other contents [56].

Thus, when removing infected tissue, the Er: YAG laser would be deactivated if changes in fluorescence are detected, indicating that all carious tissue has been removed.

Nevertheless, it is important to point out that this technique also has its limitations, as false positives can occur, due to the presence of pigments in the affected or tertiary dentin, which can distort the signal received. For this reason, a combination of manual instruments is always necessary to ensure safe and selective clinical removal of carious lesions [56].

2.4. Bactericidal effect

In addition to ablation selectivity, Erbium lasers have a bactericidal effect. Indeed, the transformation of incident radiation energy into heat leads to the vaporization of water within the bacteria, thus destroying them [71].

Authors such as Hibst et al. in 1996, reported that bacteria below the surface irradiated with the Er: YAG laser (2940 nm), are killed during cavity preparation at a depth of 300 to 400 μ.

Furthermore, it has been reported in the literature that cavity preparation with an Er, Cr: YSGG laser at output powers of 0.75 and 1W and a repetition rate of 20 Hz resulted in a statistically similar disinfectant potential to that of a chlorhexidine gluconate-based disinfectant solution (at 2%) at the cavity walls [82].

Baraba et al. in 2018, conducted an in vitro study with the aim of evaluating the efficacy of eliminating cariogenic bacteria from infected dentin with two Er: YAG lasers :

- *Fluorescencefeedback controlled Er: YAG* laser *(FFC)* (A combination of diagnostic device and Er: YAG laser).
- Er: YAG laser based on *variable* square pulse *(VSP)* technology, which works at different pulse durations: super-short SSP, short-medium MSP and short pulse SP [11].

The authors also studied the temperature rise at pulpal level during the removal of carious tissue by these two lasers.

The result of this study was in favor of complete elimination of cariogenic bacteria (Gram-positive and Gram-negative) in all experimental groups, without causing excess temperatures that could harm pulpal vitality.

Nevertheless, it has been reported that temperatures measured in groups of teeth irradiated with VSP technology during caries removal were significantly higher than those in the FFC group [11].

2.5. Ablation speed and treatment duration

The major disadvantage of Erbium lasers is the longer time required for caries treatment and cavity preparation, compared with conventional burr treatment.

Indeed, authors such as Keller et al. in 1997 and Celiberti et al. in 2006 have shown that the Erbium laser takes almost 2.5 times longer than a turbine milling cutter to prepare cavities of similar size.

Sarmadi et al in 2018, concluded at the end of a randomized clinical trial involving 25 patients (aged 15 to 40), with at least two carious lesions, one of which was excavated using a turbine milling cutter and the other using the Er: YAG laser, that the average time for removal of carious tissue by the Er: YAG laser was 3 times longer (13min) than that by the turbine rotary milling cutter (4min) [80].

A meta-analysis was carried out by Li et al. in 2019, systematically evaluating the applications of Er: YAG lasers for dental caries removal and cavity preparation in children [49].

The result of this study indicated that the time required by the Er:YAG laser for caries removal and cavity preparation was longer than that of the conventional mechanical method.

However, the authors pointed out that it was difficult to accurately determine the extra time required for the Er: YAG laser compared with the conventional handpiece, since it is dependent on cavity size and the practitioner's experience [49].

Tao et al. in 2017 reported that several factors can affect the speed of ablation of dental tissue by Erbium lasers such as patient age (treatment of deciduous teeth was faster than permanent teeth), caries site (occlusal caries is removed faster than proximal face caries), caries stage and different energy parameters used [85].

In addition to these factors, ablation speed was also affected by the angle of incidence of the laser beam in relation to the tooth.

Moreover, authors such as Laria et al. in 2011, have advocated placing the laser delivery tip parallel to the axis of the enamel prisms for better access to the inter-prismatic zone (structure with the highest water content), which significantly increases ablation speed [48].

Also, the use of manual instruments (sharpened curettes) in association with laser irradiation, could reduce laser treatment to an acceptable time [48].

3. Erbium laser and coronal restorations

3.1. Preparing surfaces for bonding

Based on a review of the literature, data concerning the bonding strength of bonding materials to Erbium laser-irradiated dental tissue are fairly controversial [55,82].

Indeed, while some authors such as Basaran et al. in 2011; Roheet and Khatavkor in 2012; Chen et al. in 2015 have described the use of Erbium lasers at low fluences as an alternative to conventional procedures for etching dental surfaces, other authors such as Takada et al. in 2015 have shown that laser irradiation, alone, is insufficient for the preparation of bonding surfaces and must be combined with 40% phosphoric acid treatment.

Studies by De Moor et al in 2010 and Moretto et al in 2011 have shown that the microstructure of the tooth surface irradiated with

Erbium lasers, with its irregular appearance, lack of Smear Layer and open dentinal tubules, optimizes the adhesive properties of dentin and improves the bonding quality of restorative materials compared with conventional preparation methods.

An in vitro study by Roheet and Khatavkor in 2012, the aim of which was to compare the effects of conventional acid etching with those of the Er:YAG laser (in non-contact mode) on enamel surface modifications, revealed that the latter used at appropriate parameters (75 mJ, 15 Hz) can result in a micro-retentive surface similar to that etched with 37% orthophos- phoric acid [38] (Figure 7).

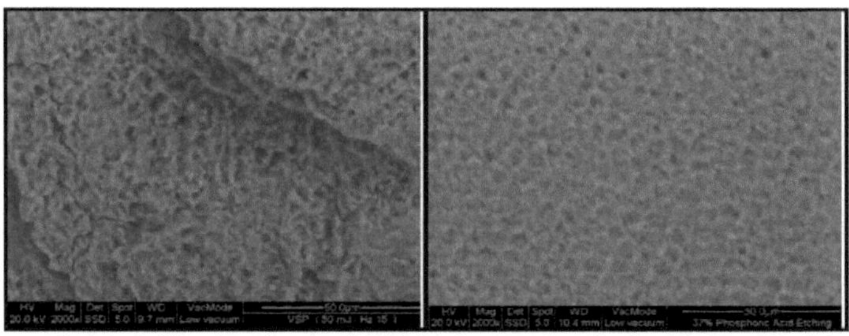

Figure 7: Magnification image (2000x) of enamel etched with Er: YAG laser (left) at 75 mJ /15 Hz and 37% Orthophosphoric acid (right)[40].

The authors thus concluded that the Erbium laser can be used as an alternative to traditional etching procedures for certain advantages: [40]

- Provides a micro-rough, debris-free surface with no smear layer.
- Antibacterial properties.
- Avoids the taste of orthophosphoric acid, which may not be well accepted by patients.

Also, Chen et al. in 2015 compared, in vitro, the efficacy of low-fluence Er: YAG laser pretreatment (150mJ; 1.5 W; 10Hz) of irradiated dentin with that of 37% phosphoric acid applied for 15s [20].

They observed that both pre-treatment methods resulted in improved bond strength between the self-etching adhesive and irradiated dentin. However, the authors reported that low-fluence Er: YAG laser irradiation offers several advantages over acid conditioning:

- The operation is more convenient and less technically sensitive than acid pre-treatment, which involves application and washing steps lasting at least 30s.

- Low-fluence irradiation sterilizes dentin tissue and reduces the risk of secondary caries.
- The Er:YAG laser has desensitizing properties that can be maintained even 6 months after the initial irradiation.

Thus, the authors concluded that Erbium laser conditioning at appropriate parameters, could be effective for composite resin bonding [20].

A systematic review of the literature was carried out by Silva et al. in 2019, the aim of which was to determine the most suitable adhesive system and laser parameters for bonding composite resin to Er, Cr: YSGG laser-prepared dentin [81].

The study involved three different self-etching adhesive systems: Adper™ Single Bond, Single Bond™ and Clearfil ™ SE.

Data from this review showed that the self-etching adhesive system (Clearfil ™ SE) showed the best adhesion results to Er, Cr : YSGG laser-irradiated dentin after 40% phosphoric acid pretreatment.

With regard to laser parameters, a setting of the Er, Cr: YSGG system at 2W, 75% water, 60% air, 140μs and 20 Hz showed the best adhesion result [81].

So, despite the arguments in favor of using Erbium lasers to prepare bonding surfaces in enamel and dentin, clinical studies are still required to observe the clinical behavior of adhesive restorations made with these lasers.

3.2. Removal of faulty restorations

Erbium radiation can easily interfere with composite resins and glass ionomer cements [82].

Indeed, given their water content, these materials have been shown to absorb Erbium wavelengths. (Keller and Hibst 1991)

Yassaei et al. in 2015, demonstrated that the Er: YAG laser generates less heat when removing adhesive materials than turbine milling cutters [89].

Amasyali et al. in 2019, conducted an in vitro study with the aim of comparing the effect of three adhesive removal methods on enamel surface roughness and dental pulp temperature [4].

The three methods used were: aluminum oxide milling cutters, the Er: YAG laser (250 mJ and 4 Hz) and a tungsten carbide milling cutter.

The results of this study showed that aluminum oxide burs produced the smoothest enamel surface, while the Er: YAG laser produced the roughest surface.

In terms of pulp temperature rise, both types of burr (tungsten carbide and aluminum oxide) generated more heat than the Er:YAG laser during adhesive removal.

On the other hand, the literature review showed that, following its interaction with the laser beam, the composite resin explodes, solidifies and forms aggregates around the tip of the laser fiber, thus limiting its integrity.

Thus, tips altered by resin fragments must be rapidly cleaned and polished using rotating discs mounted on low-speed handpieces [71].

With regard to amalgam, Riccardo Poli et al. in 2017 suggested that this silver-based material could absorb Erbium laser energy and increase in temperature, resulting in thermal damage to the teeth and periodontal tissues [71].

In addition, amalgam melting and the release of mercury vapour can occur during laser irradiation.

For example, it has been reported that Erbium lasers are not recommended for the removal of defective amalgam or metal alloy restorations [71, 82].

► ***Clinical case illustrating caries eviction and surface preparation for Er: YAG laser bonding :***

Clinical case treated by Dr Antonis Kallis and published in 2014 in the journal "Laser and Health Academy". [38]

❖ **Case presentation**

A 35-year-old woman in good general health consulted us for cold-induced tooth sensitivity.

❖ **Investigation and diagnosis**

Clinical examination revealed 4 defective composite resin

restorations and two decayed teeth.

The most clinically sensitive tooth was 46, with an old coronal composite resin filling (Figure 8).

The diagnosis was a recurrence of caries on 46.

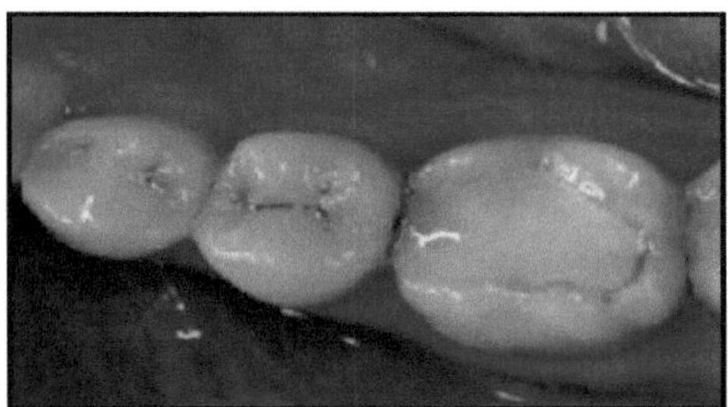

Figure 8: Preoperative clinical situation of patient 46 with a defective composite resin restoration. [38]

❖ **Therapeutic decision :**

Removal of the old composite resin restoration, curettage of the residual carious lesion and preparation of the bonding surfaces with the Er:YAG laser (Light Walker ATS, Fotona).

❖ **Operating protocol :**

➢ *Removal of old restoration: (Figure 9)*

The Er: YAG laser (2940 nm) was set to the following parameters: 1000mJ/

2 Hz in MAX mode.

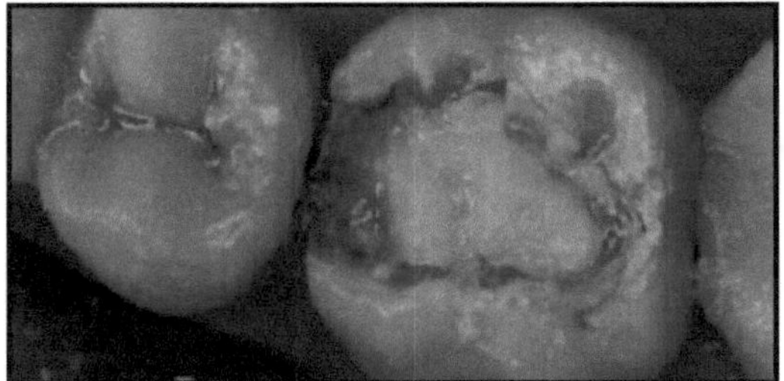

Figure 9: Removal of the old composite resin restoration. [38]

> *Curettage of residual carious lesion: (Figure 10)*

Parameters used: 200 mJ/ 10 Hz in QSP (Quantum Score Pulse) mode.

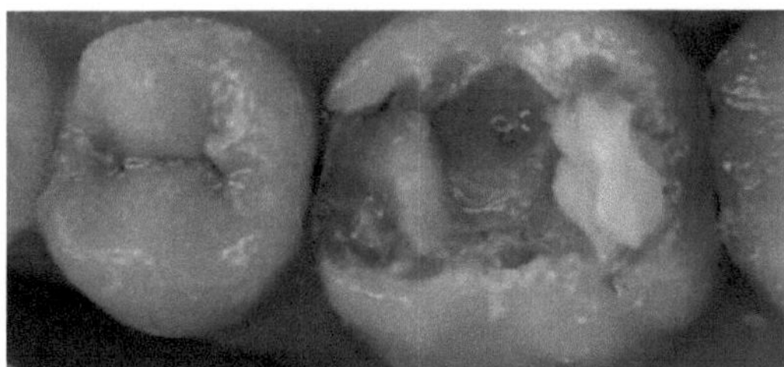

Figure 10: Ablation of carious tissue with the Er: YAG laser. [38]

The caries cavity was very deep, with bleeding in the interdental area, which necessitated the use of an Nd: YAG laser (1064 nm, 5W, 30Hz, 100 µs) to ensure hemostasis (Figure 11).

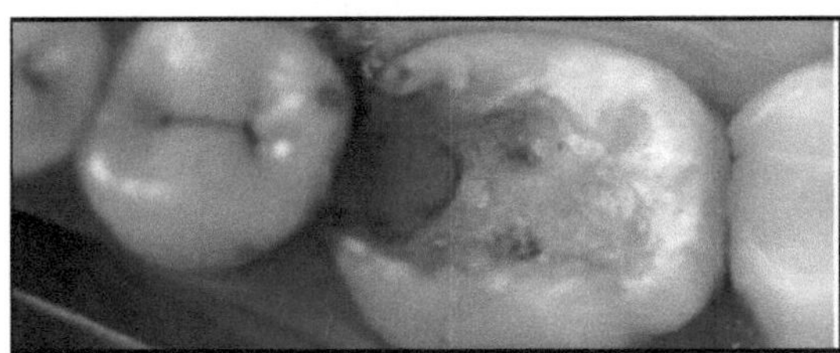

Figure 11: Hemostasis with the Nd:YAG laser. [38]

> *Preparing tooth surfaces for bonding :*

Er:YAG laser irradiation of dentin and enamel with the following parameters: 120 mJ, 10 Hz in QSP mode and without the use of acid conditioning (Figure 12).

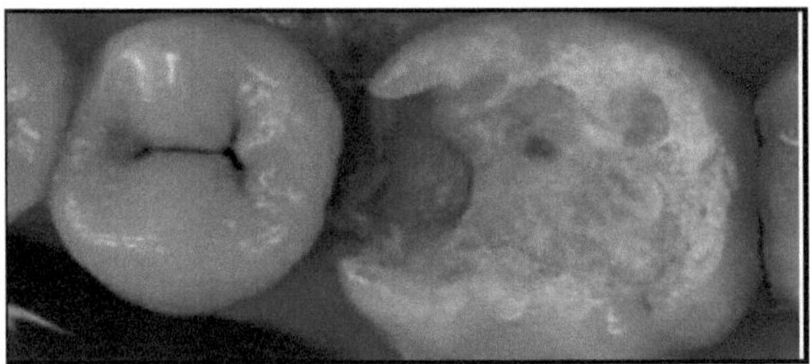

Figure 12: Er: YAG laser etching. [38]

> *Bonding of composite resin and restoration of 46 (Figure 13).* 45 was prepared using the same procedure [38].

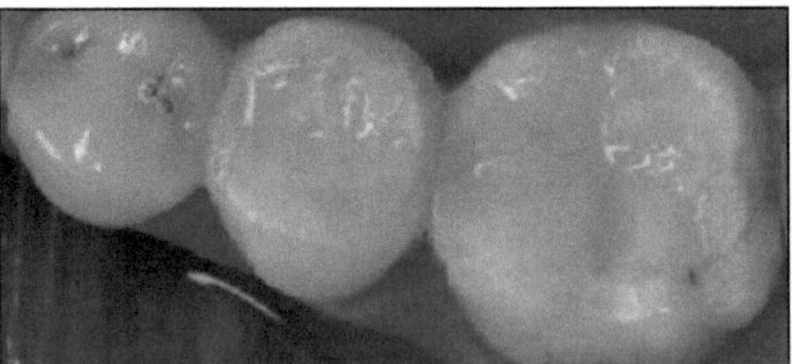

Figure 13: Postoperative view after composite resin restoration [38].

4. Dental desensitization with Erbium lasers

Nowadays, the treatment of dental hypersensitivity is considered a real challenge for professionals, as no desensitizing treatment tried in recent years has been very effective in terms of therapeutic effect and duration of action. (Aranha et al.2011)

One of the most recent forms of treatment is dental desensitization using LASER-assisted treatment [17].

Indeed, several authors such as Yilmaz et al. in 2011; Aranha et al. in 2012 and Yu et al. in 2013 have shown that laser irradiation at low energy densities can cause both the evaporation of dentinal fluids and the obliteration of tubuli by dentinal fusion, thus minimizing tooth hypersensitivity.

A randomized, controlled, double-blind clinical study conducted by Aranha et al. in 2012, with the aim of evaluating the efficacy of both Er: YAG (2940 nm) and Er, Cr: YSGG (2780 nm) lasers in the treatment of dental hypersensitivity, showed that both lasers, used at sub-ablative parameters, were able to significantly reduce pain levels in patients immediately after irradiation and over a 4-week period [6].

Similarly, Yilmaz and Bayindir in 2014 conducted a randomized controlled clinical trial with the aim of evaluating and comparing the desensitizing and occluding effects of the Er, Cr: YSGG laser on dentinal tubules with different power settings [90].

The study involved 20 patients (60 teeth).

For each patient, the teeth were randomized into 3 groups:

- Group 1 and 2: treated with the Er, Cr: YSGG laser at 0.25W and 0.5W, respectively.
- Group 3 (control): the same laser was applied without laser emission (placebo effect).

Dentine hypersensitivity was assessed for all groups using a visual analog scale (VAS).

The clinical results of this study were in favor of a significant and immediate reduction in dentine sensitivity by Er, Cr: YSGG laser irradiation with the two output powers used.

However, laser irradiation at 0.5W showed better dental desensitization results immediately after treatment: the VAS scores of group 2 (0.5W) were significantly lower than those of group 1 (0.25W). SEM observation confirmed this clinical result, as dentinal tubule diameters of teeth irradiated at 0.5W power were smaller than those irradiated at 0.25W (Figures 14 and 15).

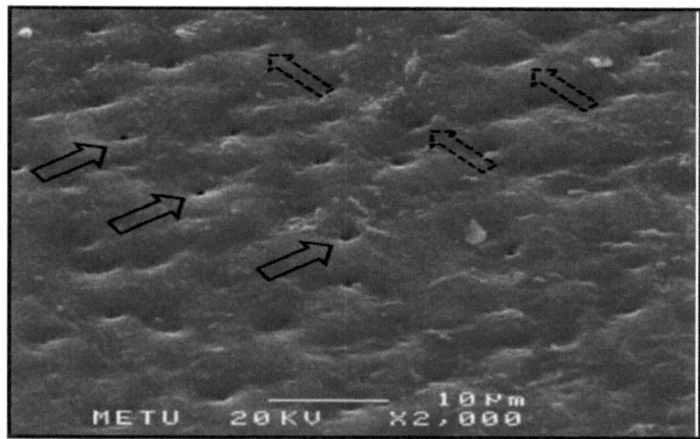

Figure 14: SEM observation of dentin irradiated with Er, Cr : YSGG laser at 0.25W. Black arrows show partially obliterated tubules and dotted arrows show completely closed tubules. [90]

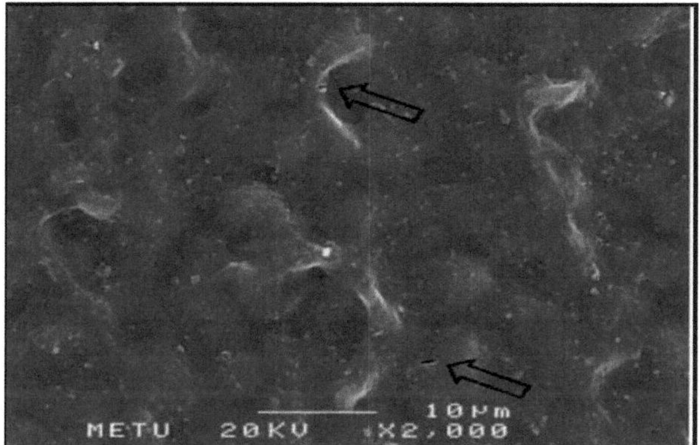

Figure 15: SEM observation of dentin irradiated with the Er, Cr : YSGG laser at 0.5W showing a significant reduction in dentinal tubule diameters. [90]

For their part, Ozlem et al. in 2018 conducted a clinical study with the aim of comparing the efficacy of a desensitizing agent containing glutaraldehyde(GCA), an Nd: YAG laser, an Er, Cr: YSGG laser and their combination (desensitizing agent-laser) in reducing dentine hypersensitivity over a 6-month period [67]. The study involved 17 adult patients with 100 teeth with dentine hypersensitivity; the patients were randomly divided into 5 groups according to the treatment protocol:

- Group 1: Application of GCA to sensitive teeth.
- Group 2: Irradiation of sensitive teeth with Nd:YAG laser ($1W/cm^2$, 10Hz).
- Group 3: Application of GCA to sensitive teeth, followed by Nd:YAG laser irradiation.
- Group 4: Er, Cr: YSGG laser irradiation ($0.25W/cm^2$, 20Hz).
- Group 5: Application of GCA to sensitive teeth, followed by

Er, Cr laser irradiation: YSGG.

Sensitivity measurements were performed using the "Yeaple" probe (pressure-sensitive electronic probe) on the vestibular surfaces of the teeth after 30 min, 1 week, 3 months and 6 months of treatment.

At the end of this study, the authors reported that a significant reduction in dentine sensitivity was observed in all tooth groups. However, the Er, Cr: YSGG laser with or without application of the desensitizing agent was the most effective in the treatment of dentine hypersensitivity [67].

Thus, the literature review showed that Erbium laser irradiation could be a promising treatment for dentine sensitivity. However, further studies are needed to assess the long-term effects of this technique, as well as the ideal laser parameters for improved dentinal tubule occlusion.

Erbium lasers (Er: YAG and Er, Cr: YSGG) in endodontics

1. Direct pulp capping

Laser irradiation of exposed pulp was first described by Moritz et al. in 1998, using a carbon dioxide laser (CO_2) to stimulate dentine bridge formation.

Since then, various laser systems, including Erbium lasers (Er; YAG and Er, Cr: YSGG), have been suggested for direct pulp capping due to the many effects they provide [45].

► Hemostatic and coagulant effect

Compared with traditional haemostasis techniques (cotton soaked in haemostatic agent), lasers can quickly and effectively stop pulpal bleeding by sealing blood vessels [45].

However, the diode laser (980 nm), which has a relatively high penetration depth into biological tissue, was more effective in terms of hemostasis than Erbium lasers (Olivi et al in 2007).

► Decontamination effect

Non-contact Erbium laser irradiation preserves the asepsis of exposed pulp tissue [45].

► Biostimulation effect :

The use of low-energy lasers can stimulate the proliferation, migration and cytodifferentiation of odontoblastic cells, thereby promoting the formation of reparative dentin in the pulp cavity. (Eduardo et al in 2008)

A meta-analysis was conducted in 2016 by Deng et al. with the aim of evaluating the effects of LASER on the outcome of direct pulp capping [25].

Of 510 studies identified, five were included, involving 4 different laser systems. The results of these studies are detailed in the following table: (Table N°IV)

Table IV: Results of the study done by Deng et al. in 2016. [25]

The study	Laser type	Pulp capping materials	Follow-up time	Success rate in laser group	Success rate in control group
Moritz et al, 1998 (24,78)	Dioxide Carbon	$Ca(OH)_2$	2 years	93%	68%
Moritz et al, 1998 (11,24)	Carbon Dioxide	$Ca(OH)_2$	1 year	89%	68%
Olivi et al, 2007 (24,52)	Er,Cr :YSGG Er : YAG	$Ca(OH)_2$	4 years	77%	75%
Yazdanfar et al, 2015 (2,24)	Diode	Resin-modified glass ionomer cement	1 year	100%	60%
Cengiz and Yilmaz, 2016 (24,61)	Er, Cr: YSGG	$Ca(OH)_2$ Light-curing liner based on resin-modified calcium silicate.	6 months	100%	70%

At the end of this meta-analysis, the authors concluded that LASER significantly improves the prognosis of direct pulp capping compared with conventional methods. Indeed, the success rate of laser groups in all studies was higher (89.9%) than that of control groups (67.2%), with a statistically significant difference (P<0.0001).

Cengiz et al in 2016 conducted a randomized clinical trial with the aim of evaluating the efficacy of Er, Cr: YSGG laser combined with calcium hydroxide $Ca(OH)_2$ or a resin-modified tricalcium silicate-based material (TheraCal LC®) in direct pulp capping, for a 6-month follow-up period [19].

The study involved 60 permanent teeth from 60 patients between the ages of 18 and 40 with exposed pulp and no clinical symptoms or radiological damage. The teeth were randomly divided into 4 groups, each of which received a different pulp treatment:

Group 1: The exposed pulpal area was sealed with $Ca(OH)$ paste$_2$.

Group 2: The exposed area was sealed with calcium hydroxide after irradiation with an Erbium Er, Cr: YSGG laser at a power of 0.5W without water sprays.

Group 3: TheraCal LC was applied directly to the pulp wound.

Group 4: TheraCal LC was applied after Er, Cr : YSGG laser irradiation.

The results of this study showed that the success rates for the $Ca(OH)_2$ and TheraCal groups were 73.3% and 66.6% respectively, while for both Laser groups the success rate was 100%.

Thus, the authors concluded that, Er, Cr: YSGG laser irradiation at 0.5W and in combination with pulp capping agents can be recommended for direct pulp therapy [19].

According to Komabayashi et al. in 2016, the protocol for direct pulp capping with lasers (CO_2, Nd: YAG, Er: YAG, Er, Cr: YSGG and diode laser) includes the following steps: [45] (Figure 16)

- Anaesthesia (unless pain).

- Placement of the operating field (dike).

- Complete curettage of the decayed dentine surrounding the pulp opening using rotary instruments, taking care not to further damage the exposed pulp.

  Erbium lasers are also recommended for removing carious tissue and preparing cavities, as they prevent thermal damage to pulp tissue.

- Hemostasis and decontamination of the pulp wound: The advantage of using the laser at this stage lies in its non-contact mode, which preserves the asepsis of the exposed pulp.

- Placement of capping material after hemostasis has been achieved.

- Tight coronary restoration.

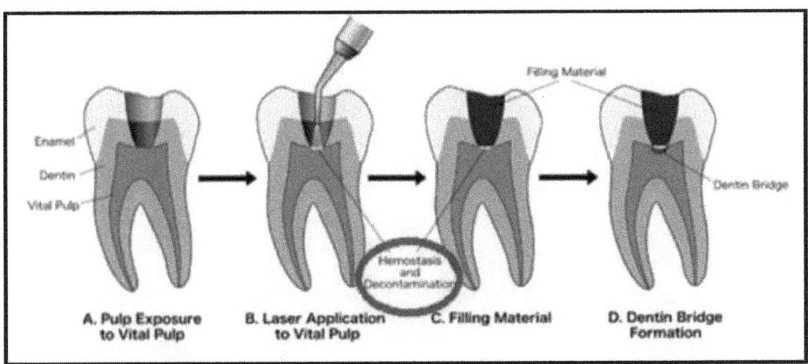

Figure 16: Direct laser pulp capping protocol. [45]

▶ *Clinical case illustrating Er: YAG laser pulp styling :*
Clinical case treated by Dr Pawel Roszkiewicz and published in 2017 in the Journal "Laser". [76]

❖ **Case presentation**

A 35-year-old patient presented to the clinic with a deep site 2 carious cavity (Occluso-Mesial) on the 16th. Due to the complexity of the cavity and in order to avoid pulpal exposure, the bottom of the cavity was partially cleaned and then covered with two types of non-hardening (UltraCal™ XS) and self-hardening (Ultra-Blend®) calcium hydroxide. The cavity was then filled with a temporary obturation material.

The patient reported no pain, and sensitivity to stimuli was similar to that experienced in other maxillary molars.

❖ Explorations and Diagnosis

In order to assess the extent of pulpal damage to the tooth and its chances for biological treatment, a retroalveolar radiograph of 16 was taken. (Figure 17)

The X-ray suggested (red arrow) the presence of calcifications in the pulp chamber.

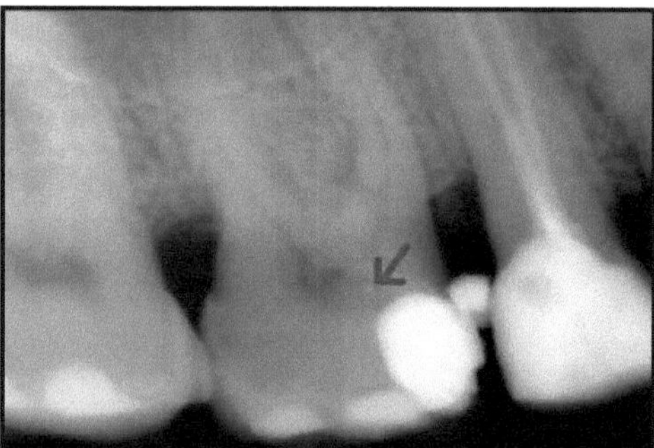

Figure 17: Preoperative radiograph of 16 [76].

❖ Therapeutic decision

- Reconstruction of the mesial wall with composite resin.
- Use of the Er:YAG laser (Light Walker, Fotona) for hemostasis and cavity disinfection.

- Direct pulp capping of 16 with Biodentine™ followed by composite resin restoration.

❖ **Operating sequence**

- Local anesthesia.
- Removal of part of the temporary ultrasound dressing to create the space needed to reconstitute the mesial wall and position the operating field (dam).
- Cleaning was continued with the Er: YAG laser (Light Walker, Fotona), using the H14 contact contra-angle handpiece with a 1.3 mm diameter cylindrical optical fiber, placed approximately 1 mm from the tooth surface.
- The laser parameters used during cavity preparation are shown in Table 9.
- Reconstruction of the mesial wall of 16 with composite resin.
- Installation of the dike.
- Removal of the entire temporary dressing using ultrasound: pulp exposure of 1 to 1.5 mm in diameter was revealed, with a delicate effusion of a colorless, odorless liquid that stopped after 2 to 3 min, confirming the theory of pulp hyperemia in response to the application of calcium hydroxide (Figure 18).

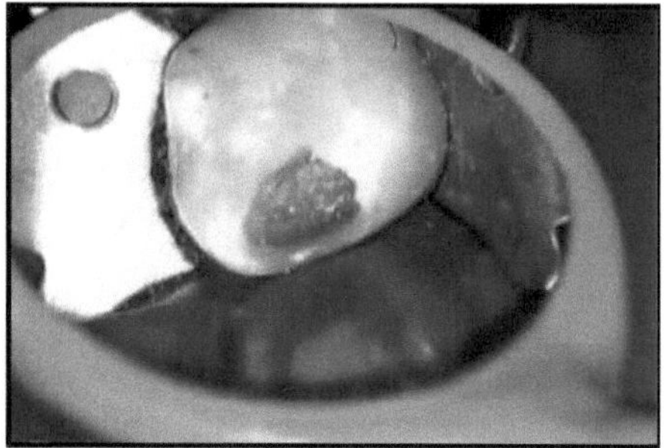

Figure 18: Pulpal exposure after cavity floor removal [76].

- In order to minimize thermal damage to pulp tissue, preparation of the deepest part of the cavity was carried out using the Er:YAG laser with reduced parameters compared to the initial preparation (Table V).

- Once the dentin surface had been cleaned, the inner surface of the filling was smoothed using a turbine diamond bur.

- Removal of a calcium hydroxide fragment previously pressed into the pulp chamber using a manual endodontic instrument (Figure 19).

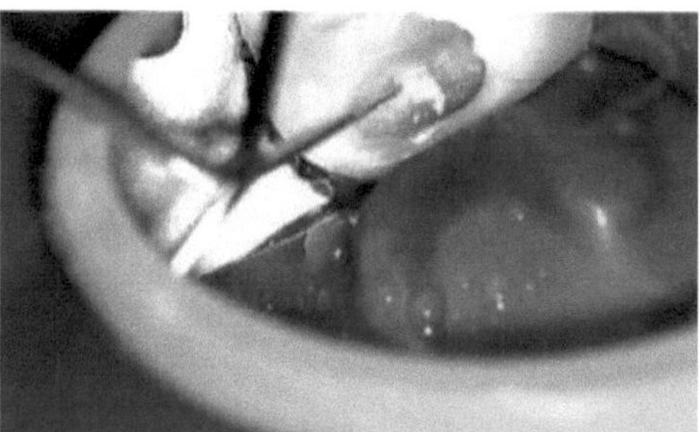

Figure 19: Removal of the calcium hydroxide fragment. [76]

- Hemostasis and disinfection: application of the Er: YAG laser (100mJ, 4Hz) at the pulpal exposure, placing the tip 5 mm from it to reduce radiation intensity (Figure 20).

The parameters used are shown in Table V.

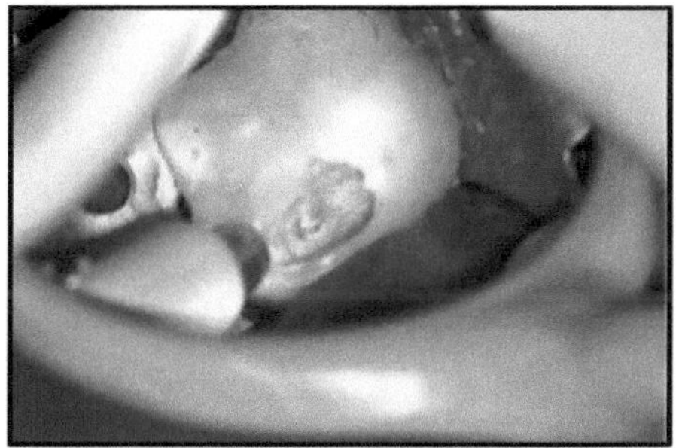

Figure 20: Hemostasis and disinfection of the pulp wound using the Er: YAG laser. [76]

- Placement of Biodentine™ to cover pulpal exposure.

    (Figure 21)

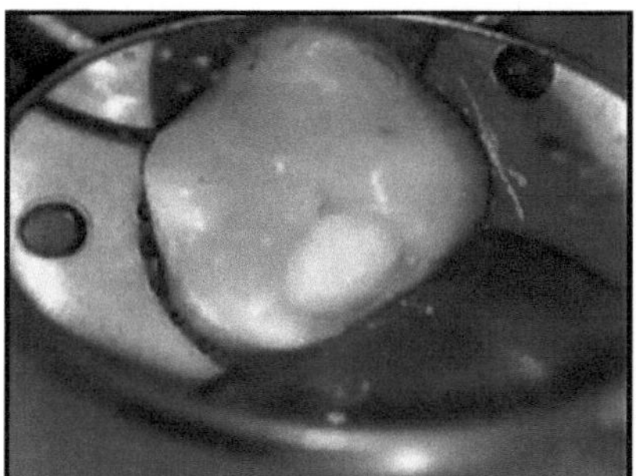

Figure 21: Pulp capping with Biodentine™ . [76]

- After Biodentine™ has set, restore the tooth with the composite resin previously used to build up the mesial cavity wall (Figure 22).

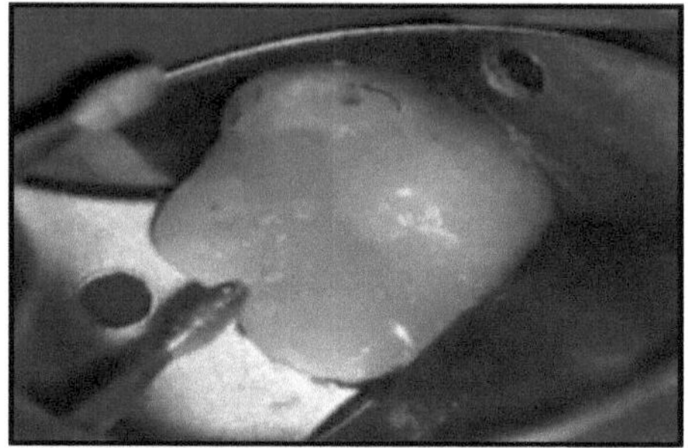

Figure 22: Coronal restoration with composite resin. [76]

■ Postoperative control radiograph (Figure 23).

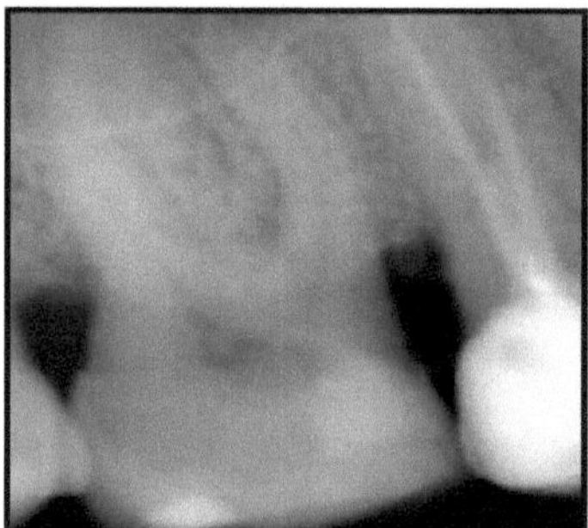

Figure 23: Postoperative follow-up radiograph. [76]

Table V: Er: YAG laser parameters used during treatment. [76]

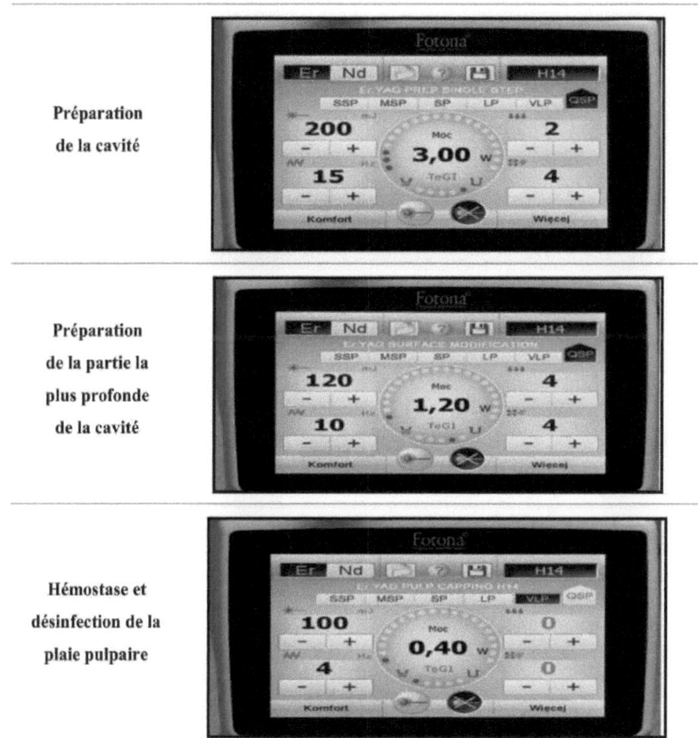

Préparation de la cavité	
Préparation de la partie la plus profonde de la cavité	
Hémostase et désinfection de la plaie pulpaire	

2. Preparing access cavities

In addition to the conventional use of rotating instruments, access to the pulp chamber can be achieved using Er: YAG (2940nm) and Er, Cr: YSGG (2780 nm) lasers.

The literature review showed that, for this stage of endodontic treatment to be successful, Erbium lasers need to be set to the right parameters.

Divito et al in 2012, recommended the use of a short optical fiber (4 to

6 mm) with diameters of 600 to 800 micrometers, made of quartz to enable the use of high energies and powers [30].

Olivi et al in 2016, showed that the use of degressive energy from dentin to pulp over the course of access cavity preparation enables effective and safe ablation of hard and soft dental tissues [65].

In fact, the high affinity of Erbium lasers with carious tissue and pulp (both rich in water) means they can both curettage decayed dentine and progressively uncover pulp horns with lower energy, thus reducing the risk of misdirections.

The authors recommend using the following energy values, depending on the tissue concerned [65] (Table VI).

Table VI: Erbium laser energy values as a function of target tissue. [65]

Fabric	Email	Decayed dentine	Pulp	Channel inputs
Energy	250 mJ	150 mJ to 200 mJ	150 mJ	80 mJ to 120 mJ

In an earlier study, Mazeki et al. (2003) evaluated the effectiveness of the Er:YAG laser in preparing root canal orifices on 36 extracted human teeth (in vitro) and on 11 teeth from 11 patients with irreversible pulpitis (in vivo) [58].

For the in vitro study, parameters of 250 mJ / pulse and 8 Hz were used, with an irradiation duration of 60s for monoradiculated teeth and 120s for pluriradiculated teeth.

However, in the clinical study, the energy of the Er:YAG laser was reduced (160 mJ/pulse; 8Hz) for greater ablation safety.

The results of this study showed:

- In vitro: root canal orifices of 31 out of 36 teeth (86%) were successfully exposed without rim formation or perforation.

- ■ In vivo: root canal orifices of 10 out of 11 teeth (91%) were successfully prepared, and no rim or perforation formation was observed.

The authors concluded that the use of Erbium lasers for root canal exposure can be effective, if the appropriate parameters are respected.

On the other hand, it has been reported in the literature that Erbium lasers enable a considerable reduction in bacterial load as access cavities are prepared, thus reducing the transport of bacteria, toxins and debris apically during root canal preparation [26,30,65].

According to Cheng et al in 2012, during Laser-assisted access cavity preparation, bacteria will be destroyed to a depth of 300 to 400 microns from the irradiated surface.

Erbium lasers can also be used to remove pulpolites and find the canal entrances of calcified canals [30].

Despite their advantages, there are several recognized limitations to the use of Erbium lasers for the preparation of endodontic access cavities, namely [65] :

- ■ The time required for preparation is rather slow.
- ■ Lack of control over the stripping of the access cavity walls.
- ■ The difficulty of eliminating all dentinal overhangs without risking perforation.

2. Root canal shaping

Canal preparation using Nickel-Titanium instruments is now the benchmark technique in endodontics. Indeed, despite the recognized ablative effect of Erbium lasers (2780 nm and 2940 nm) on hard tissue, their effectiveness in root canal shaping appears limited at present, and does not match the endodontic standards achieved with NiTi instrumentation.

However, some studies have reported favourable results concerning the effectiveness of Erbium lasers in shaping and widening root canals [43,60].

Inamoto et al in 2009 observed morphological changes in root surfaces irradiated with Er:YAG lasers using SEM.

They reported that the latter were well cleaned, with no debris or "Smear Layer" dentinal sludge, and with well-opened dentinal tubules. Also, no pulp residue was detected after irradiation (Figure 24).

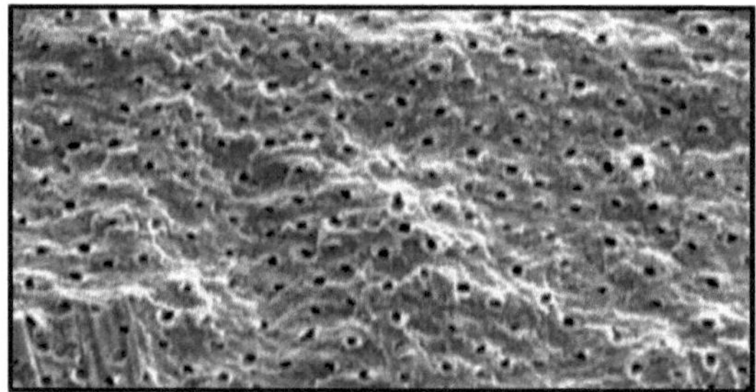

Figure 24: SEM observation of Er:YAG laser irradiated root dentin (magnification×1000) [36].

Minas et al in 2009, compared the enlargement to the correct working length, the amount of dentinal sludge and the opening of dentinal tubules of canals prepared conventionally (endodontic files) and others prepared with the Er, Cr: YSGG laser (2780nm) using the Step-Back technique [59]. The study involved 15 extracted posterior human teeth (with multiple canals), with zero or minimal curvature (<12°).

The tooth canals were explored to ensure their permeability and radiographed to determine the exact working length (WL) using K files; ISO sizes 10 and 15.

The final TL was set at 1 mm from the apical foramen.

The laser used in this study was set to an output power of 2W and a frequency of 20 Hz, with 50% air pressure and 50% water.

Channel shaping with the Er, Cr: YSGG laser in contact mode and with the Step-Back technique was carried out according to the following sequence:

- Widen the apical portion of the canal with K files (10, 15 and 20), up to ISO diameter 20, to allow insertion of the smallest 200µm Z2 tip (corresponds to ISO diameters 20 and 25).
- Insert 200µm tip at working length and activate laser.
- Hold the tip in the apical zone for 2s, then withdraw in a coronal direction parallel to the canal walls at a speed of 2mm/s.
- Insert 320µm (ISO 35) Z3 tip at LT-3mm and handle in the same way.
- Insertion and handling of the latest 400µm Z4 tip (ISO 40-45) at LT-4mm.

During the procedure, the canals were constantly moistened with water and were not irrigated with any endodontic irrigation solution.

For conventional debridement, the canals were prepared conventionally with K files, using the Step-Back technique, up to the ISO diameter of the master apical file 30 with additional flaring up to ISO diameter 40-60.

A 2.5% NaOCL irrigation solution was used after each file pass, and a complete canal wash was performed with saline at the end of preparation.

At the end of this study, the authors found that it was possible to prepare canals using the Step-Back technique, using laser irradiation with specific fiber tips, however, conventional debridement had a higher success rate than laser (80% vs. 60%) [60].

Similarly, Roper et al. in 2010 compared the conventional method of root canal preparation using rotating NiTi instruments (ProFile®) with that assisted by the Er: YAG laser (2940 nm), measuring the amount of dentin removed in different sections of root canals [75].

They showed that the two techniques were equivalent in terms of cleaning and debridement of the canals in the coronal and medial thirds. However, the conventional technique was more effective in preparing the apical third.

Also, the authors reported that the laser took almost twice as long to clean the canals as the conventional method [75].

In 2012, Kokuzawa et al. evaluated in vitro the ability to shape the apical portion of the canal using an Er:YAG laser equipped with tapered fibers of 185 and 280 microns in diameter; the tapered fibers scattered 80% of the laser energy laterally.

Irradiation was performed at 0.4 W (20 Hz, 20 pulses/s) with water spray (5ml/min), 3 times for 10s.

SEM observations showed a clean dentin surface with open tubular orifices.

However, irradiation with the 280 micron fiber resulted in more root dentin ablation than the 185 micron fiber.

The authors pointed out that laser ablation efficiency was inversely proportional to the square of the distance between the laser fiber and the canal walls. Thus, it was suggested that the degree of cutting could be increased by using a laser fiber adapted to each stage of debridement [43].

On the other hand, the literature has reported that root canal surfaces prepared with Erbium lasers, although well cleaned and free of "smear layer", often contain ledges, irregularities and carbonization with a high risk of perforation or apical transport [30].

Furthermore, Olivi et al. in 2016 reported that root canal shaping with Erbium lasers, remains a complex procedure that can only be performed in wide, straight canals [65].

3. Activated irrigation and bactericidal action

According to Paque et al in 2011, adequate diffusion and penetration of antibacterial irrigation solutions in the root canal network is still necessary to promote debridement and disinfection of the canals.

However, traditional root canal irrigation (syringe and needles) often fails in this respect, as significant numbers of bacteria remain in the canals even after abundant irrigation (Boutsioukis et al. 2009; Zehnder et al. 2012).

Various irrigation activation techniques have been proposed in the literature to improve the distribution and efficiency of irrigation solutions in the root canal system. These include dynamic manual activation, hydrodynamic activation, ultrasonic activation and sonic activation [65].

One of the most recent techniques for irrigant activation in the root canal is laser-activated irrigation, combining chemical irrigation and laser irradiation with the aim of optimizing intracanal debris removal and minimizing bacterial load [65].

Two techniques for activating intracanal irrigation with Erbium lasers have been presented in the literature: "LAI" *(Laser Activated Irrigation)* and "PIPS" *(Photon-InducedPhotoacoustic Streaming).*

IPM is a global term, and PIPS is a specific IPM technique performed with the Er:YAG laser.

4.1. Activation of Erbium Laser Irrigation (LAI)

▶ LAI's mechanism of action

The bactericidal effect of IPM is based on the principle of cavitation: the photons excited in the root canal system by the Erbium laser encounter the water molecules in the irrigation solution (generally sodium hypochlorite), causing these molecules to implode by sublimation, forming a water plasma. This plasma reaches a temperature of 1500°C over a period of a few microseconds in the pulp chamber. The water contained in the root canal system turns to steam and creates bubbles, which grow and increase the pressure of the liquid in the pulp chamber and then in the root canal network.

These bubbles join together, increase in volume and then explode, generating high pressure in the fluids.

The increase in pressure, coupled with the explosion of water molecules, generates a violent shockwave which will promote the bursting of bacterial membranes and the removal of dentinal debris from canal walls [14,57].

▶ Operating protocol

Once canal shaping is complete, the canal is filled with irrigant, and the optical fiber is inserted 1 mm from the working length. Four to five series of shots are fired in a back-and-forth motion, and the irrigant solution is renewed each time (Figure 25) [44].

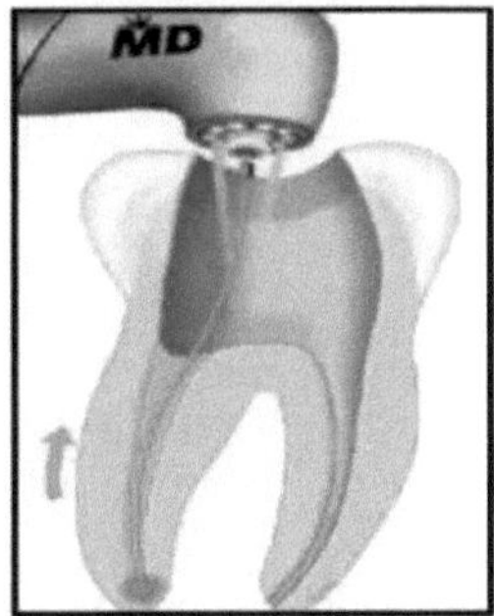

Figure 25: Schematic representation of the IPM technique. [44]

Two irrigation solutions have proven their effectiveness in the LAI procedure, given their strong absorption in the Erbium wavelengths: [30,86]

■ Sodium hypochlorite (NaOCL): used in various concentrations (2.5% to 6%), it has a bactericidal action.

What's more, the increase in temperature during irradiation with Erbium lasers potentiates the bactericidal effect of sodium hypochlorite insofar as it enables a more rapid release of chlorine; one minute of NaOCL laser activation is equivalent to 3 minutes of non-activation. (Marcedo et al. in 2010)

■ Ethylene Diamine Tetraacetic Acid (EDTA 17%): Has a

chelating action that helps eliminate dentin sludge.

Thus, for the LAI technique, successive washes of 17% EDTA followed by sodium hypochlorite, interspersed with applications of laser irradiation, are recommended for at least 10s for each irrigant [26].

With regard to the laser parameters used during IPL, the literature review showed considerable variation in pulse energies (between 20 and 80 mJ), pulse frequencies (from10 to 35 Hz), pulse duration (between 50 and 130µs) and laser irradiation time (from 5 to 40s) [59]. Variations in laser fiber tip diameter (from 200 µm to 600 µm), shape (flat or conical) and position in the channel have also been reported in the literature [30,65].

Meire et al. in 2016, reported that the best results for root canal debris removal by LAI were observed when the Er: YAG laser fiber was introduced into the canal, 2mm from the LT, and used with the following parameters: a short pulse duration of 5µs, a pulse energy of 40 mJ, a frequency of 20 Hz, during a long irradiation time (from 20 to 40s).

In contrast, the same authors reported that fiber shape and diameter had no statistically significant influence on LAI efficacy [59].

On the other hand, the laser activation technique requires ISO 25 or ISO 30 root canal preparation in order to insert the smallest 200µm laser fiber at root canal level [30,44].

▶ **Role of LAI in root canal decontamination**

In an in vitro study in 2015, Sahar-Helft et al. compared the efficacy of three irrigation techniques in removing the Smear Layer from canal walls: positive pressure irrigation, passive ultrasonic irrigation and laser-activated irrigation [77].

They reported, following SEM observation of the root dentin surface, that removal of the dentin sludge layer was more effective when the root canals were irrigated using the LAI technique with the Er: YAG laser set at low energies (0.5W, 50 mJ, 10Hz).

In addition, the authors reported that the result was similar when the laser was inserted in the coronal third of the canal or 1 mm from the LT. In fact, the removal of dentin sludge in the laser groups involved the entire canal wall (from the coronal third to the apical third), with dentin tubuli wide open along the entire length of the canal. This was not the case with syringe irrigation, where dentin sludge was still present in the apical third of the canal, and with ultrasonic irrigation, dentin tubules were partially closed in this apical zone (Figures 26 and 27).

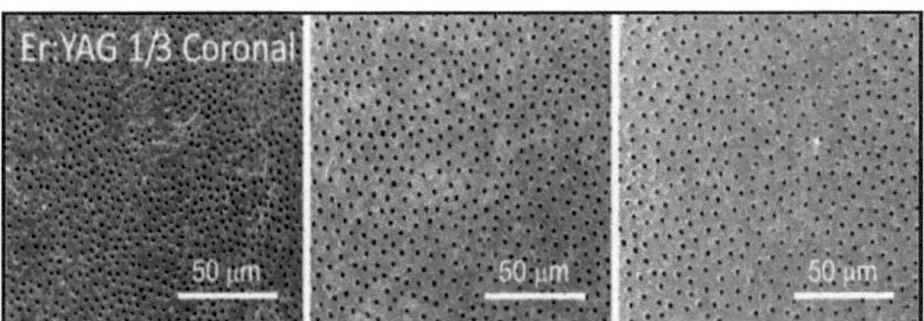

Figure 26: SEM observation of the coronal (left), medial (center) and apical (right) parts of the root canal wall. LAI with 17% EDTA and laser tip inserted in the coronal part of the root canal (magnification × 1000) [77].

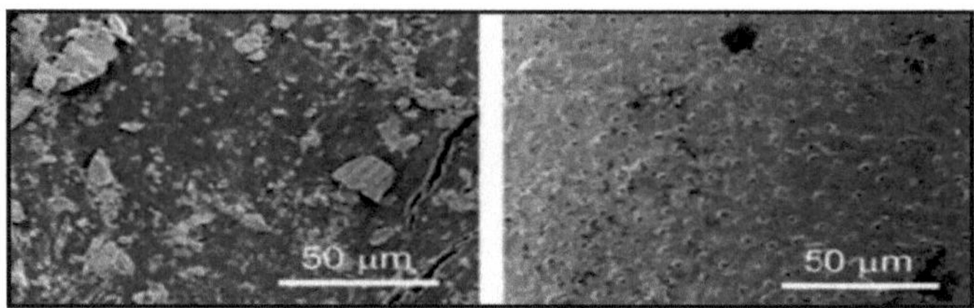

Figure 27: SEM observation of the apical part of the canal walls. Syringe irrigation (left); ultrasonic irrigation (right). (Magnification × 1000) [77]

Wang et al in 2017, evaluated in vitro the efficacy of Erbium laser-activated irrigation (Er: YAG and Er, Cr: YSGG), in combination with two irrigation solutions: NaOCL (5.25%) and EDTA (17%) in removing the dentin sludge layer from canal walls [87].

They found, after SEM observation, that activating irrigation potentiated the decontamination effect of irrigants at root canal level.

Nevertheless, it was reported that the protocol combining the LAI technique with both irrigants (EDTA and NaOCl) was more effective than that using the same technique with a single irrigation solution.

Kihara et al. in 2019 showed that Er: YAG laser-activated irrigation (30mJ, 20 Hz, 100µs, without water or air cooling) of a 5% NaOCL solution for 20 or 40s more effectively removed gelatin hydrogel (used as a substitute for root canal debris) from a simulated accessory canal than conventional syringe irrigation.

However, the authors reported that LAI for 40s removes, significantly, more hydrogel than in 20s (P<0.05) [41].

Concerning its bactericidal effect, several authors such as De Groot et al., 2009; Zhu et al.,2013; Cheng et al., 2016, have reported the effectiveness of Erbium laser irrigation activation in eliminating the bacterial biofilm of Enterococcus Faecalis (E. Faecalis), which is the most virulent bacterium in the endodontic system.

Indeed, due to its numerous virulence factors (presence of surface proteins, aggregating substances, filaments, etc.), this bacterium is very often resistant to conventional irrigation solutions and intracanal medication, thus increasing the failure rate of root canal treatment. (Fisher et al., 2009) Moreover, given its ability to survive in conditions normally lethal to other micro-organisms: a highly saline environment (6.5% NaCl), basic pH, high temperature (60°C), and in the presence of detergents, this bacterium is one of the main causes of secondary endodontic infections and outbreaks (Stuart et al., 2009).

Cheng et al. in 2017, revealed that the Er: YAG+NaOCl combination, was able to reduce the bacterial load of E. Faecalis biofilm by up to 98.8% compared to conventional syringe irrigation (94%) [22].

Wang et al. in 2018 compared, in vitro, the bactericidal effect of various irradiation systems on Enterococcus faecalis biofilm in dentinal tubules: conventional irrigation with NaOCL 5.25% (1ml), Nd:YAG laser irradiation (1064nm), Diode laser irradiation (980 nm), Nd:YAP laser irradiation (1340nm), Er, Cr:YSGG laser LAI with NaOCL (5.25%) and Er:YAG laser LAI with NaOCL (5.25%) [88].

They demonstrated that Erbium laser-activated irrigation for 3 min had the strongest bactericidal effect of all the protocols tested, with root canal disinfection rates reaching 85% for Er, Cr: YSGG+NaOCL and 89% for Er: YAG+NaOCL.

3.1. Photon-Induced Photoacoustic streaming (PIPS)

PIPS is an acronym first described by Enrico DiViti in 2006 and stands for photon-induced photoacoustic scattering.

This is a specific activated irrigation technique that uses the Er: YAG laser (2940nm) and relies on the interaction of the photons generated with the water molecules contained in the endodontic irrigation solutions [37].

This interaction differs from that of the LAI technique in that it is based on a photoacoustic rather than a photothermal phenomenon (no vaporization of the solution).

▶ **PIPS mechanism of action**

Unlike conventional laser applications, the fiber does not need to be placed in the canal, but only in the pulp chamber, and is used in a stationary manner (Figure 28) [37,65].

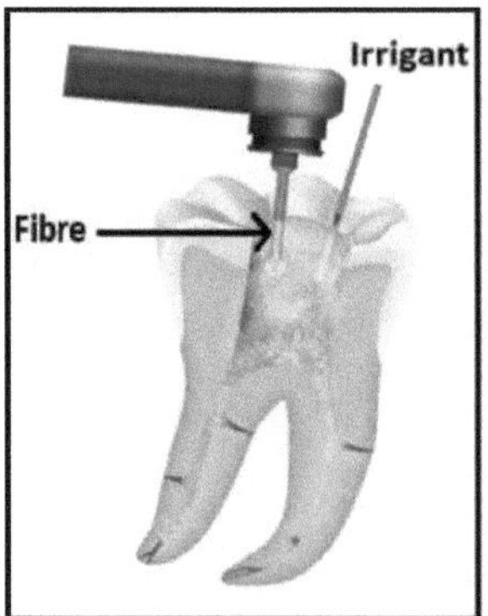

Figure 28: Illustration of the PIPS technique. [65]

The high absorption of the Er:YAG laser wavelength by the irrigant solution, combined with a 400W pulse at the tip, generates successive expansive photoacoustic waves. This phenomenon drives the irrigant through the root canal system [30].

PIPS operates at sub-ablative energies (20mJ to 50mJ) and high pulse powers (400W to 1000W) [65].

It uses a specific fiber: a quartz fiber (600µm, 9mm) with radial emission and a stripped end over its last four millimeters (Figure 29).

The advantage of this fiber is that it emits less energy at its tip with a stripped part, improving the lateral distribution of energy [65].

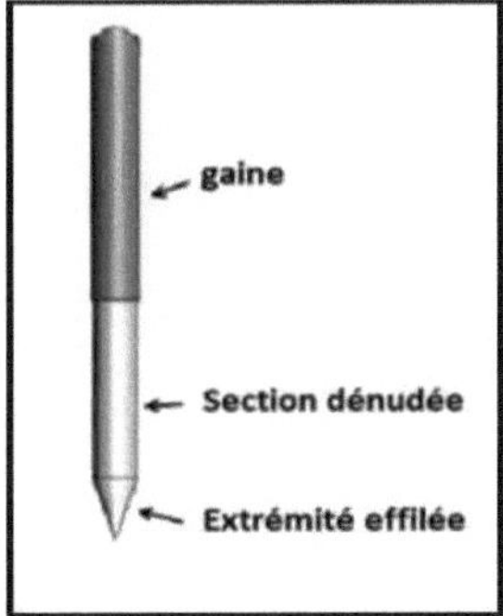

Figure 29: Schematic representation of the fiber used in PIPS. [65]

▶ Operating protocol

A major advantage of using PIPS is that it enables non-invasive endodontic treatment that does not require excessive enlargement of the canals for insertion of the optical fiber (the fiber is placed higher in the pulp chamber) [30].

David Jaramillo et al. in 2015 established a PIPS clinical protocol (Figure 30) [37].

The PIPS technique is performed instead of the traditional final rinse at the end of root canal preparation. However, Deponte in 2018 reported that this technique can also be used during the root canal shaping stage between the passage of two endodontic instruments [26].

The PIPS protocol itself: (Figure 30)

The Er: YAG laser is set to 20 mJ; 15Hz and with spray deactivated.

- 3 cycles of 30s PIPS activation with continuous flow of NaOCL (5%) and 30s rest between each cycle.

- 30s PIPS activation with a continuous flow of distilled water.

- 30s PIPS activation with continuous flow of EDTA (17%).

- Final rinse by laser activation of distilled water for 30s.

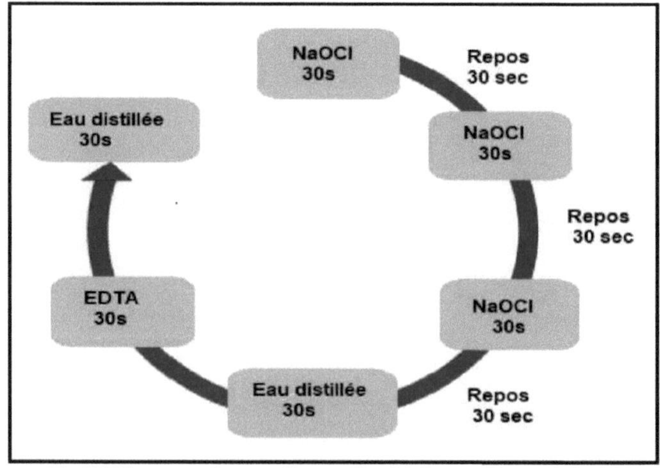

Figure 30: PIPS protocol according to David Jaramillo et al. in 2015. [37]

▶ PIPS and root canal disinfection

Olivi et al in 2014, conducted an ex vivo study on 26 human anterior teeth with the aim of comparing the efficacy of root canal disinfection using PIPS with the conventional irrigation method [65].

Teeth were prepared to ISO 25 size, then infected with Enterococcus faecalis and incubated for 4 weeks.

The authors used two irrigation protocols.

Group "A" received two 30s cycles of laser activation of 5% NaOCL solution (3ml) and one 30s cycle of 17% EDTA activation (3ml).

Er: YAG laser settings were 20mJ, 15Hz and a short pulse duration of 50µs.

Group "B" received two 30s cycles of conventional irrigation (using a syringe) with 5% NaOCL (3ml), followed by a 30s cycle of 17% EDTA (3ml).

Both groups were irrigated with distilled water for 30s after each irrigant, to avoid any chemical reaction between the two irrigation solutions.

The results of this study showed:

- Immediately after treatment: bacterial reduction of 99.99% and 99.83% for groups A and B respectively.
- 48h after treatment: bacterial reduction was 99.99% in group A, but no reduction in group B (0%).

The authors found that both irrigation techniques were effective in eradicating E. Faecalis biofilm from canal walls. However, PIPS had a more persistent effect (48 h after treatment), inhibiting new bacterial growth [65].

Golob et al in 2017, evaluated in vitro the effect of varying NaOCL concentration (1%, 3% and 5%) on the efficacy of PIPS in root canal disinfection [32].

For effective smear layer removal, the authors modified the sequence and resting time of the final PIPS irrigation steps.

The modified irrigation protocol was as follows:

1. Activate 3 ml NaOCL for 30s, then rest for **60s**.

2. Activate 17% EDTA for 30s, then rest for **60s**.

3. 2 activation cycles of 3 ml NaOCL of 30s each, interspersed with a **60s** rest period.

4. Activate 3ml distilled water for 30s.

This study showed that :

- Decontamination of the canal network was effective and long-lasting only when 5% NaOCL was used. In the groups treated with 1% and 3% NaOCL, bacteria returned to the canals 48 hours after treatment.

- The modulus of elasticity and flexural strength of dentin depend on the concentration of NaOCL: during instrumentation, irrigation with 3% NaOCL was most recommended to avoid weakening of dentin and erosion of dentin surfaces.

- Applying EDTA prior to NaOCL cleans the dentin surface and opens the dentinal tubules, thus promoting the penetration and bactericidal action of NaOCL on the E. Faecalis biofilm.

The authors found that laser-activated irrigation of 5% NaOCL, together with the modified PIPS protocol, resulted in effective eradication of bacterial biofilm and complete elimination of the smear layer [32].

The literature also reports the effectiveness of the PIPS technique in removing calcium hydroxide (inter-session root canal medication) from root canal walls.

Arslan et al. in 2015 compared, in an in vitro study, the effect of activating a 17% EDTA irrigation solution for 60s using different techniques, on the removal of $Ca(OH)_2$ from artificial grooves along the canal wall [8].

The result of this study showed that PIPS removed 100% calcium hydroxide, in contrast to ultrasonic activation (76%) and manual syringe irrigation (25%).

Furthermore, Aricioglu et al. in 2018, using the same irrigation conditions (17% EDTA for 60s), showed that none of the irrigation techniques used (PIPS, passive ultrasonic PUI irrigation, sonic irrigation, conventional syringe irrigation) completely removed calcium hydro xyde from artificial grooves in canal walls [7].

However, these authors reported that PIPS and PUI were more effective than other irrigation methods, and that no statistically significant difference was found between these two techniques. (P>0.001)

Laky et al in 2018 advocated an Er: YAG laser parameter setting of 10 mJ/ 15Hz for almost complete (99.5%) removal of calcium hydroxide from canal walls, without apical extrusion of irrigation solution [47].

5. Definitive root canal filling

According to the literature review, laser irradiation of dental root surfaces could improve the seal of the definitive root canal filling.

Previous studies by Kimura et al. in 2001 and Sousa-Neto et al. in 2005 have demonstrated that laser treatment (Er: YAG; Er, Cr: YSGG and

Nd: YAG) contributes to the effective removal of the smear layer and the opening of dentinal tubules, thereby increasing the adhesion of sealing cements and filling materials to the canal walls.

Ayranci and Koseoglu in 2014, suggested that morphological changes in root dentin walls obtained by Er: YAG laser irradiation could influence the adhesion values of root canal sealing cements [9].

Indeed, these authors showed that the adhesion of AH Plus® (resin-based root canal cement) to the canal walls was better after Er:YAG laser treatment of root dentin, compared to other treatment methods (5% NaOCL, 15% EDTA followed by 5% NaOCL, Nd:YAG laser).

Ozkocak and Sonaten in 2015 evaluated, in vitro, the bond strength of three types of root canal sealing cements: AH Plus Jet®(Dentsply), EndoSequence BC Sealer™ (Brasseler) and Real Seal® (Sybron Endo), after irradiation of root dentin with the Er: YAG laser [66].

They showed, after SEM observation, that Erbium laser irradiation resulted in the complete elimination of dentin sludge and the opening of dentin tubules, which favoured the penetration of sealing cements into the dentin. Also, the presence of surface irregularities and micro-retentive zones after irradiation, were in favour of increasing the bond strength of the sealing cements at root canal wall level [66].

However, the authors reported that the resin-based luting cements "AH Plus Jet®" and "Real Seal®" showed higher bond values to irradiated dentin (120MPa) than the bioceramic-based cement "EndoSequence BC Sealer™" (80MPa). This difference was explained by the fact that the latter, due to its hydrophilic nature, requires the presence of water to bond to root dentin. This was not the case after evaporation of the interstitial fluid at the level of the dentinal tubules following laser irradiation [66].

Regarding the root canal obturation technique recommended after Er: YAG laser root canal shaping, Kokuzawa et al in 2012 reported that the vertical gutta percha condensation technique may be more appropriate than lateral condensation due to the irregular rough surfaces generally formed by laser irradiation [43].

In 2014, Gérard Rey et al. in their book entitled "Utilisation des lasers en endodontie" (Use of lasers in endodontics) reported on the usefulness of the Er:YAG laser in compacting gutta percha at root canal level [74].

Thanks to its dual photothermal and photomechanical effects, this laser both raises the temperature of the gutta-percha and mechanically propels it and the luting cement.

The protocol described by the authors was as follows:[74]

- Root canal filling paste (zinc oxide-eugenol) is deposited in the root canal using a paste tamp or lentulo.
- The Er: YAG laser, thanks to its photomechanical effect, can be used at this stage to propel the paste into the open tubuli; it is set at a low energy of 60 to 80 mJ and a low frequency of 5 Hz.
- A decontaminated, dried and calibrated gutta-percha cone is inserted into the canal.
- Softening of gutta-percha by photothermal action of Er: YAG laser (60mJ; 15Hz).
- Compacting the gutta using hand tools (vertical rammers).
- Propulsion of gutta percha by the photomechanical effect of the

Er:YAG laser in accessory and lateral canals.

- Manual compaction completes the procedure, to obtain a satisfactory, hermetic obturation of the root canal system.

6. Endodontic treatment

The usefulness of lasers in the endodontic retreatment procedure lies primarily in their photothermal effect, which dissolves gutta-percha and removes it from the canal walls. (Blum et al. ,2000 ; Viducic et al. ,2003)

Keles et al in 2015, in a micro-computed tomography study, evaluated the efficacy of removing root canal filling materials (Gutta-percha and AH Plus® sealing cement) by two laser systems Er: YAG (2940nm) and Nd: YAG (1064 nm) from root canal walls [39].

They showed that additional irradiation with the Er:YAG laser after root canal retreatment with rotating instruments (R-Endo®NiTi) resulted in significantly higher removal of obturation material remnants (13%) from the root canal walls than with the Nd:YAG laser (3%).

Furthermore, it has been reported that unlike the low-energy pulsed Er: YAG laser (50mJ, 20Hz), the heating effect of the Nd: YAG laser probably affected the surrounding dentin, causing it to melt and promoting the melting of leftover filling materials, thus increasing their retention to the canal walls [39].

Tachinami and Katsumi in 2010, studied in vitro the ability of the Er: YAG laser used at different output energies (30mJ, 40mJ and 50mJ) to remove root canal filling materials during endodontic retreatment [83]. The study involved 21 extracted, monoradiculated human teeth with a relatively straight canal that were obturated with gutta-percha using the lateral condensation technique.

After laser irradiation, the elements evaluated were: the time required to remove the root canal filling material, the quantity of material remaining, and the degree of root dentin removal during endodontic retreatment (degree of dentin loss from the root canal wall).

The conclusions of this study were as follows:

- The higher the laser output energy, the shorter the gutta removal time.

- Almost all the gutta-percha has been removed from the channel for all three energy groups.

- Only a small amount of root canal dentin was lost when the obturation material was removed, and there was no statically significant difference between the three energy groups.

- Irradiation at an energy of 50mJ revealed carbonization stains on the channel wall, observed under a digital microscope.

- Er:YAG laser irradiation at an output energy of 40 mJ could effectively remove gutta-percha without causing perforation of the root canal wall or excessive ablation of root canal dentin.

A study by Gorduysus et al. in 2019 evaluated the effectiveness of Er: YAG laser irradiation used at different output energies (40mJ and 50mJ) compared with ultrasound (NEWTRON® P5) in removing gutta percha during endodontic retreatment. This study revealed that the laser beam was not as effective as ultrasound in reaching the deepest parts of canals (especially the apical third), and that it also generated secondary thermal damage (burn spots and charring of dentinal tubule orifices) even at the lowest energy used (40mJ) [33].

The authors also noted that the Er:YAG laser took longer to dissolve the entire root canal filling than ultrasound: The mean time for removal of gutta percha by ultrasound was 18.71s, whereas for laser it was 77.42s (for 40mJ/pulse) and 113.57s (for 50mJ/pulse) [33].

As a result, the use of Erbium lasers in root canal retreatment procedures has so far been less reliable and cannot be considered an alternative to the retreatment methods used in our daily practice. However, the ongoing development of equipment and techniques suggests that results will improve in the future.

> ***Clinical case illustrating the contribution of the LAI technique in endodontic retreatment.***
> *Clinical case treated by Dr Sharonit Sahar-Helft and Dr Adam Stabholtz; published in 2016 in the journal "Stomatology Edu".* *[78]*

❖ Case presentation :

A 42-year-old diabetic male consulted for a fistula at the back of the vestibule in the region between 12 and 13.

The history revealed that the fistula had been present for more than 2 years.

A locating radiograph was taken with a gutta-percha cone to determine the causal tooth (Figure 31).

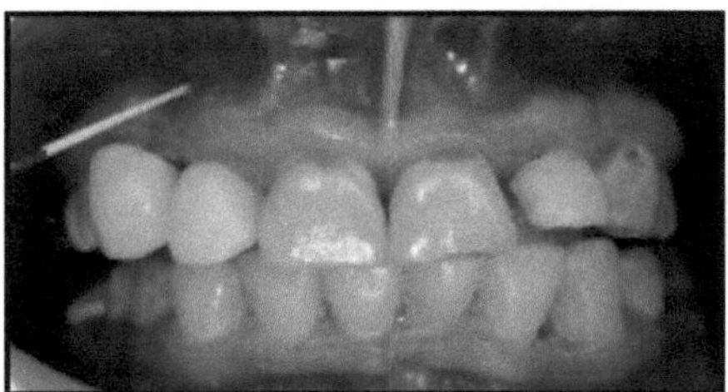

Figure 31: Preoperative photograph showing the fistula. [78]

❖ Explorations and Diagnosis

On clinical examination, 12 presented with a metal-ceramic crown. There was no pain on percussion, and periodontal probing was normal. Radiological examination revealed a periapical radiolucency image related to endodontically-treated 12. The gutta cone confirmed this relationship and also the causal tooth (Figure 32).

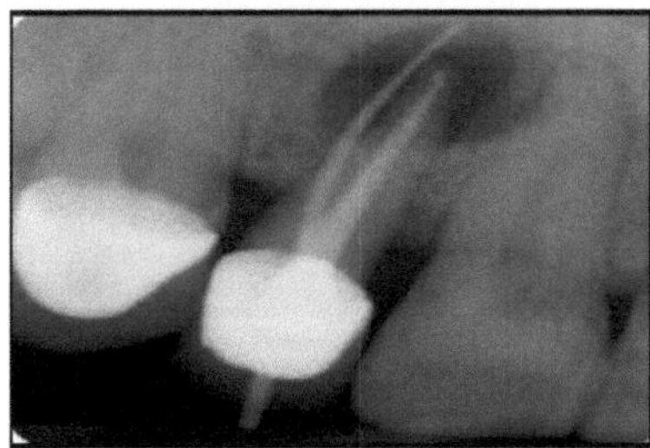

Figure 32: Spotting radiograph showing a periapical lesion related to endodontically treated 12. [78]

❖ Therapeutic decision

Crown removal on 12 for orthograde endodontic treatment.

During the cleaning and root canal shaping sessions, several intra-canal medications were used, such as calcium hydroxide, a mixture of 3 antibiotics (metronidazole, minocycline and ciprofloxacin) and Ledermix. After several sessions, the fistula persisted.

The practitioners decided to use Er:YAG laser-activated irrigation (LiteTouchTM) to optimize root canal disinfection.

❖ **Operating sequence**

■ Surgical drape in place.

■ The Er: YAG laser was activated at 50 mJ, 0.5W and 10 Hz for 60 seconds using 17% EDTA as irrigation solution. (Figures 33 and 34)

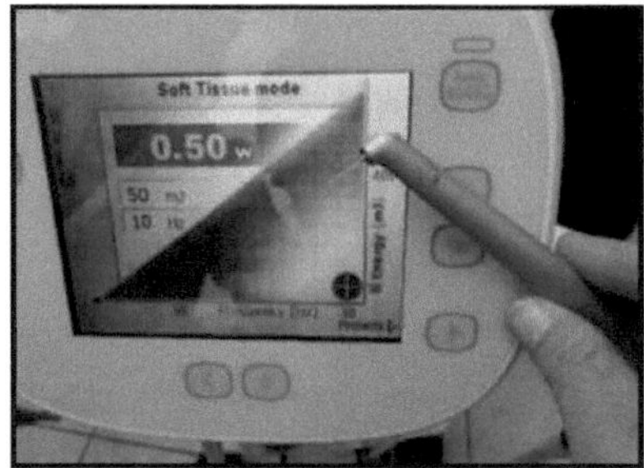

Figure 33: Er: YAG laser parameters used. [78]

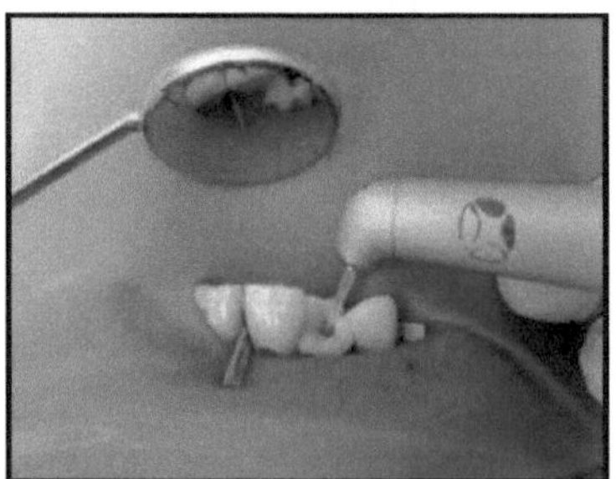

Figure 34: Er:YAG IPL procedure [78].

The final root canal filling was performed at the same session.

Approximately 2 years post-operatively, the follow-up radiograph showed complete disappearance of the periapical image and healing of the periapical tissues. (Figure 35).

Clinically, the fistula disappeared.

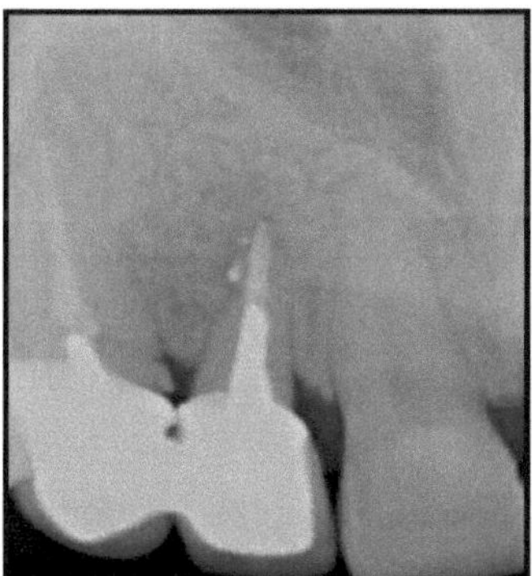

Figure 35: Control radiograph at 2 years post-operatively. [78]

7. Endodontic surgery

Erbium LASERs are of great interest in endodontic surgery.

Used in the various phases of surgical treatment (mucosal incision, osteotomy, apical resection and retrograde cavity preparation), these lasers have shown high success rates compared with conventional treatment techniques [91].

In 2011, Angiero et al. conducted a study to evaluate the efficacy of erbium lasers in retrograde endodontic treatment in terms of clinical results and therapeutic success. The study involved 65 necrotic teeth with apical lesions whose apicectomy was performed with two types of Erbium lasers: Er: YAG (2940 nm) and Er, Cr: YSGG (2780 nm) during the period between 2000 and 2010 [5].

The results of this study showed that therapeutic failure occurred in only 9 cases at different times; the other patients (86%) presented no complications, and their treatment progressed favorably.

The authors report that Erbium lasers appear to be perfectly suited to the various phases of retrograde treatment: they are equipped with very fine optical fibers (from 320µm to 600µm), they possess a bactericidal and sterilizing action on the root apex and surrounding tissue reducing bacterial infiltration within the resected root, and they do not produce secondary thermal damage.

For their part, Bodrumlu et al in 2012 showed that the Er: YAG laser set at three different pulse durations (50µs, 100µs and 300µs) could be used, with acceptable safety for apicectomy, if the associated water spray was sufficient [15].

However, it has been reported that laser irradiation with a pulse duration of 50µs appears to have the lowest temperature rise and shortest time required for apicectomy compared with the other two pulse durations [15].

Lietzau et al in 2013, conducted a retrospective clinical investigation with the aim of evaluating the efficacy of the Er: YAG laser used in conjunction with a dental operating microscope in apical surgery, compared with the conventional surgical procedure (use of burs, without microscopic control) [50].

The results of this study were as follows:

- On the first postoperative day, redness and swelling of the surgical area were significantly reduced in the laser-treated group compared with the control group (p<0.001).

- Seven days after surgery, all inflammation parameters were significantly lower in the laser-treated group (p<0.05).

- At day 180, 6 out of 41 patients in the control group were still experiencing pain and impaired function of the treated teeth, while no patient in the laser group experienced any new complaints.

The authors thus concluded that, although it requires more operating time, Er:YAG laser-assisted surgical treatment monitored under the operating microscope provides a better healing process than the conventional surgical approach [50].

Furthermore, Shabnam et al. in 2019 suggested that apical microleakage may be better prevented when apical resection is performed with the Erbium laser than with the tungsten carbide burr.

Indeed, these authors, comparing the penetration rate of a dye (methylene blue) after apical resection with the Er, Cr: YSGG laser and retrofilling with MTA to that after conventional treatment, showed that microleakage was higher in the burr-treated group of teeth (0.42 ± 0.23) than in the laser-treated group (0.20 ± 0.16) [63].

▶ *Clinical case illustrating Er: YAG laser apicectomy.*
Clinical case treated by Dr. William H. Chen and published in 2020 in the journal "Oral Health. [21]

❖ **Case presentation**

An 85-year-old female patient presented with right maxillary pain and swelling.

❖ **Investigation and diagnosis**

Clinical examination revealed that the swelling was close to the apex of 13. The latter was an abutment of an eight-unit metal-ceramic bridge from 13 to 24 (Figure 36).

The 13 was painful to percussion and palpation.

Periapical radiography revealed bone resorption around the apex of 13, with evidence of possible perforation caused by the root post. (Figure 37)

The diagnosis of acute apical abscess was confirmed.

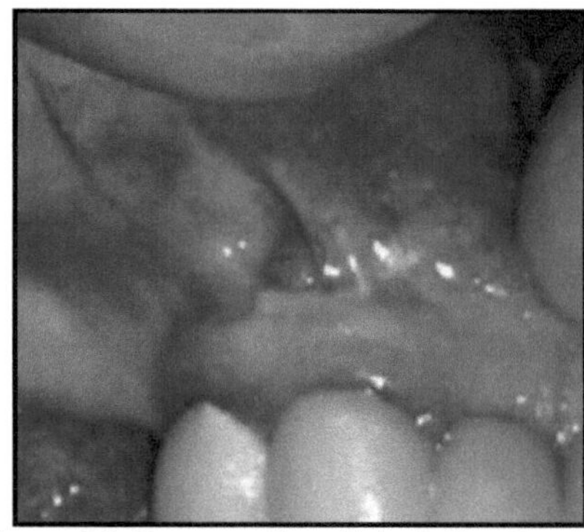

Figure 36: Preoperative clinical situation [21].

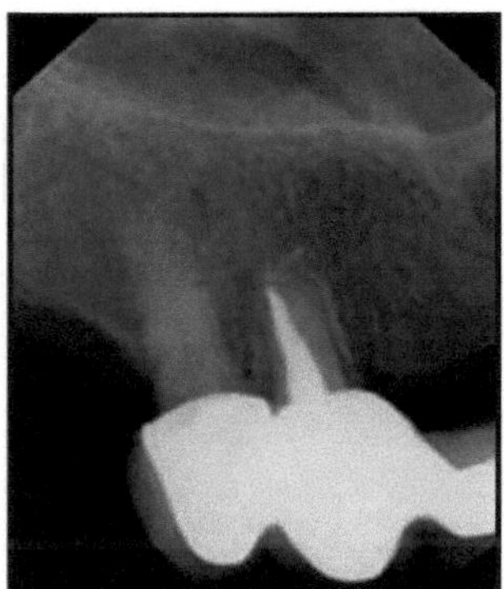

Figure 37: Periapical radiograph [21].

❖ Therapeutic decision

Since no exceptional medical or dental history was noted as a contraindication to surgical treatment, a laser apicectomy followed by retrograde obturation with MTA was programmed in order to preserve the fixed prosthesis.

The laser used is Biolase's Er, Cr: YSGG system (2780nm) with a gold handpiece and a 14mm-long MZ5 fiber.

❖ Operating sequence

- Local anesthesia of the surgical area, using two carpules of 2% lidocaine with vasoconstrictor.
- Mucogingival laser incision Er, Cr: YSGG: (Figure 38)

The laser was set at 2.5W, 30Hz, 15% water and 11% air.

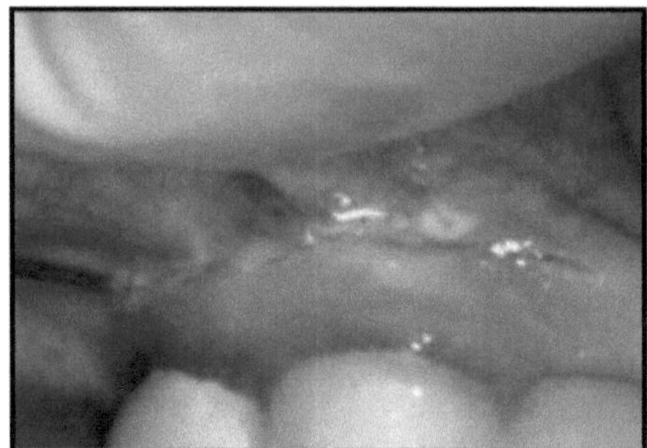

Figure 38: Mucogingival incision with Er laser, Cr: YSGG. [21]

- Removal of a trapezoidal flap using a periosteal elevator.
- Er, Cr: YSGG laser osteotomy to reveal the apical lesion and apex of 13: (Figure 39)

The laser parameters used were: 5 W, 20 Hz, 50% water and 70% air.

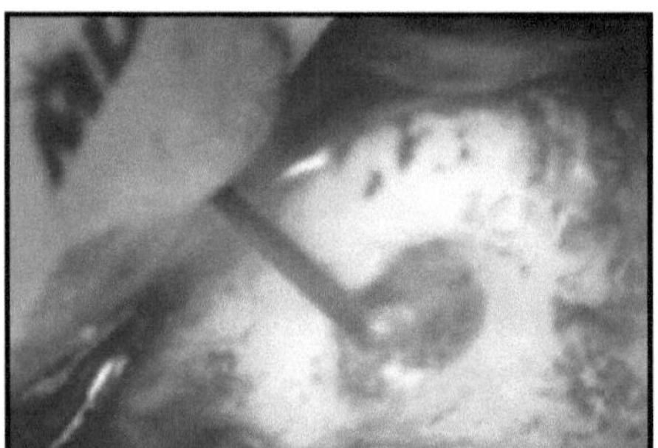

Figure 39: Er, Cr laser osteotomy: YSGG. [21]

- Granuloma removal: (Figure 40)

The Er, Cr: YSGG laser was set to 3W, 30Hz, 15% water and 11% air.

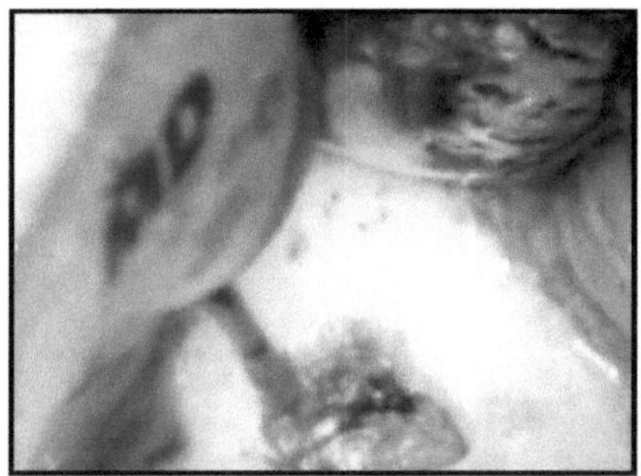

**Figure 40: Removal of granulomatous tissue with the Er, Cr: YSGG laser.
[21]**

At the end of this procedure, a few carbonization spots were revealed, due to the smaller amount of water used during granuloma removal. Also, perforation caused by the root post was noted at this stage. (Figures 41 and 42)

The carbonization stains were then removed (during final debridement of the apex and bone crypt), using the Er, Cr: YSGG laser under the "Hard Tissue" setting.

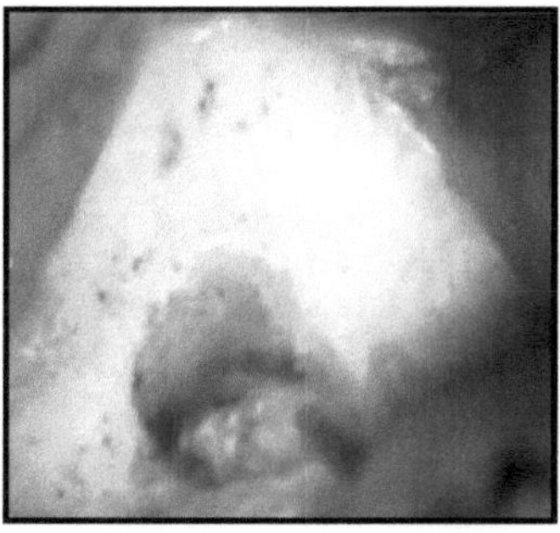

Figure 41: Appearance of charring spots at the surgical site. [21]

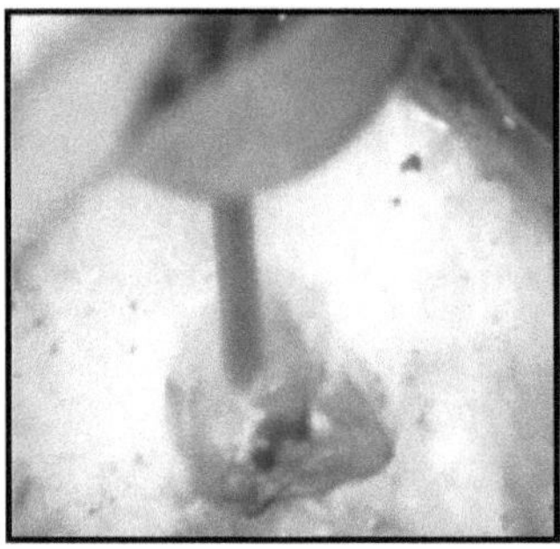

Figure 42: Root post perforation. [21]

- Removal of the apical part of the root post to allow placement of the retrograde obturation material (MTA) (Figure 43).

This step was carried out using an electric handpiece and a round stainless steel milling cutter turned at high speed.

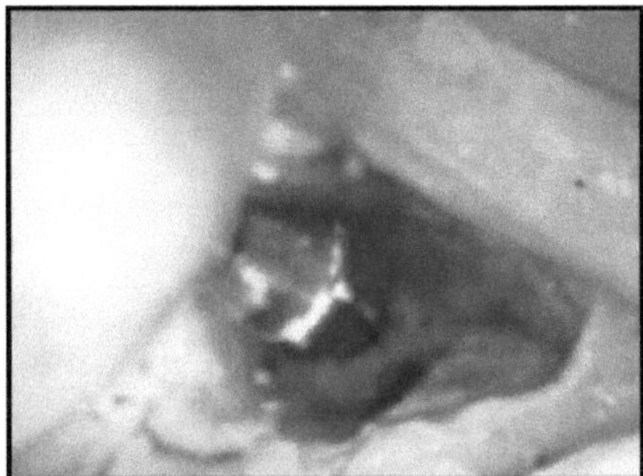

Figure 43: Removal of the apical part of the post with the burr. [21]

- Apicectomy (approx. 3 mm from root apex) with Er, Cr: YSGG laser used at 4W, 20Hz, 50% water and 70% air.
- Retrograde ultrasonic preparation: use of a Cavitron® surgical system and a Cavitron® endodontic tip (Figure 44).

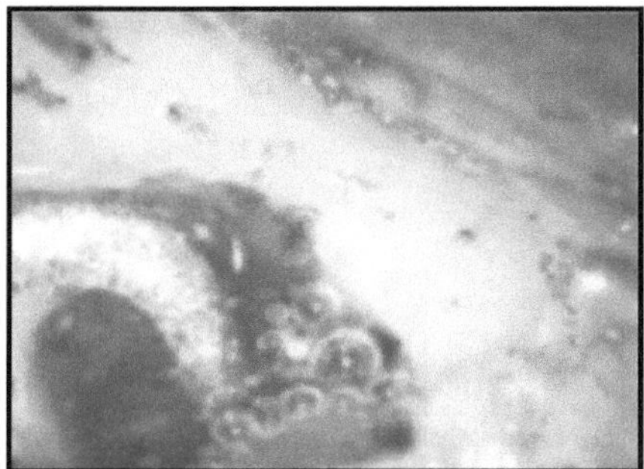

Figure 44: Ultrasound preparation of the retrograde cavity. [21]

■ Removal of the retrograde cavity smear layer with the Er, Cr: YSGG laser with the following parameters: 2W, 20 Hz, 50% water and 70% air (Figure 45).

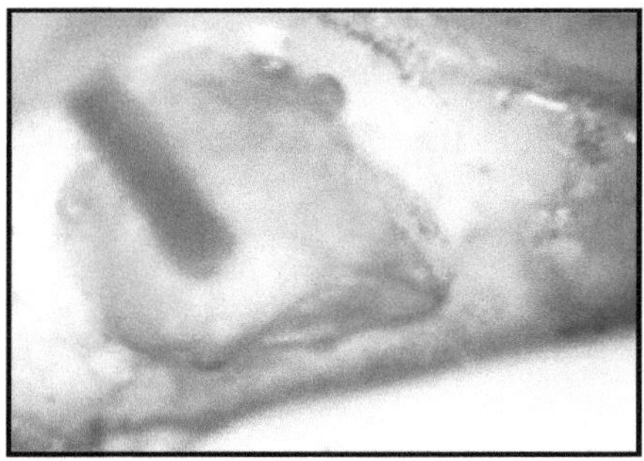

Figure 45: Smear layer removal with the Er, Cr: YSGG laser. [21]

■ Retrograde filling with MTA.

■ Suture the surgical site with Matelassier stitches using absorbable Vicryl sutures (4.0).

■ A biological "dressing" procedure was performed using the Er, Cr: YSGG laser.

This procedure consists of "Low Level Laser Therapy" aimed at hemostasis, disinfection and de-epithelialization of the surgical site. (Figure 46)

The laser setting used was 1.25W, 30 Hz, 0% water and 11 air in H mode, defocused to 5 mm and using a fast-moving laser fiber.

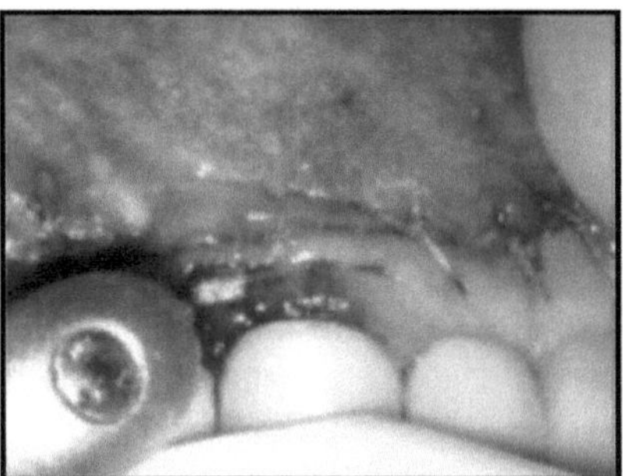

Figure 46: Biological dressing of the surgical site using the Er, Cr: YSGG laser. [21]

The appearance of the surgical site after biological dressing with the Er, Cr: YSGG laser was dry. However, the gingival tissue regained its normal color after wetting the surgical site (Figures 47 and 48).

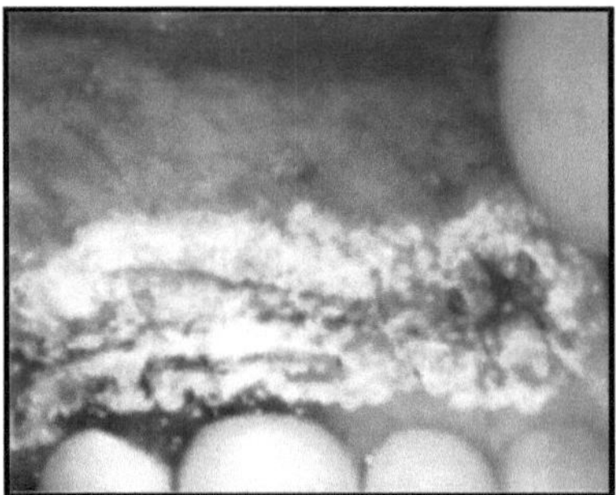

Figure 47: Dry appearance of the surgical site after the biological dressing procedure. [21]

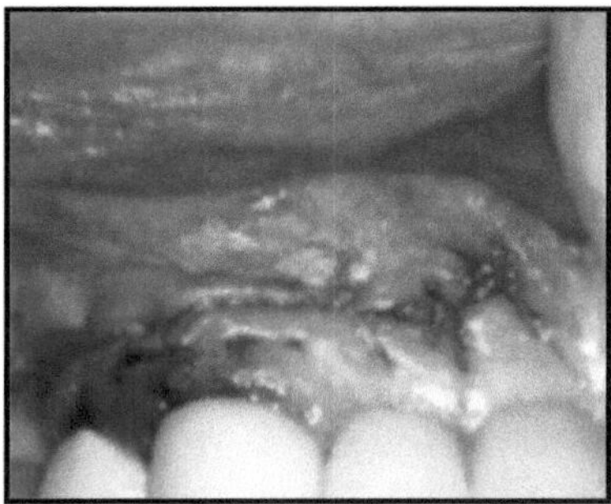

Figure 48: Immediate postoperative photograph of the surgical site. [21]

- Antibiotic and analgesic prescription.

- Post-operative recommendations were provided to the patient in the same way as those provided after tooth extraction.

The patient was given appointments for postoperative monitoring and stitch removal.

- Three days postoperatively: Clinical observation revealed that the surgical site was healing extremely well, with no signs of secondary bleeding, infection or swelling. The patient did not report or show any signs of discomfort (Figures 49 and 50).

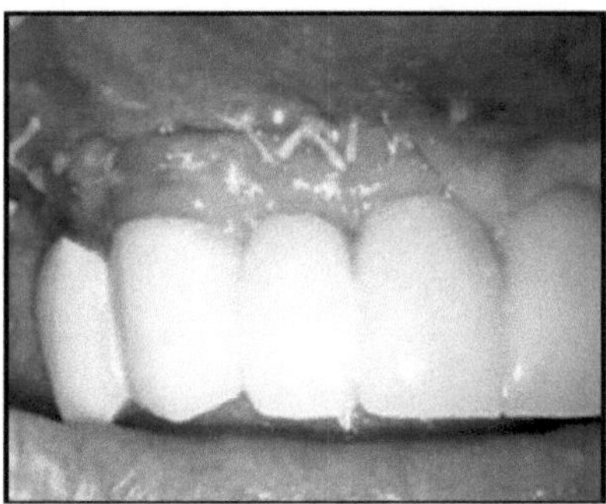

Figure 49: Clinical check-up 3 days postoperatively. [21]

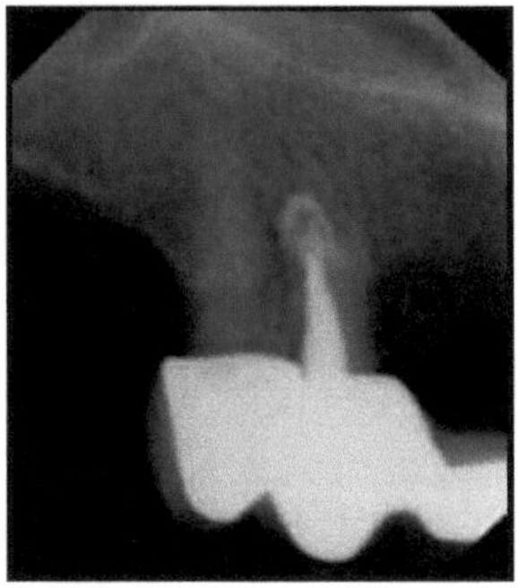

Figure 50: Radiological check at 3 days post-op. [21]

■ Three weeks postoperatively. (Figures 51 and 52)

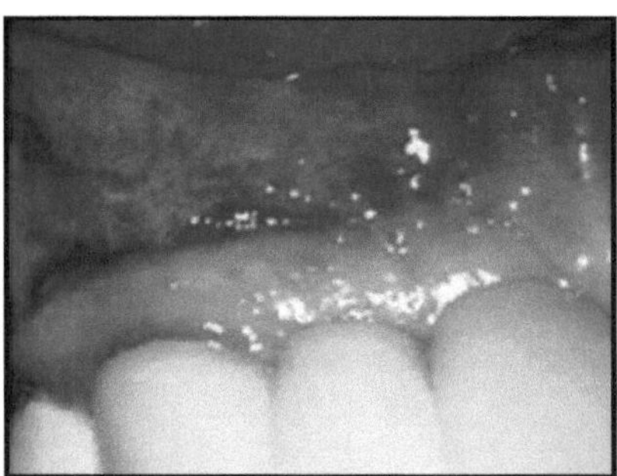

Figure 51: Clinical check-up at 3 weeks postoperatively. [21]

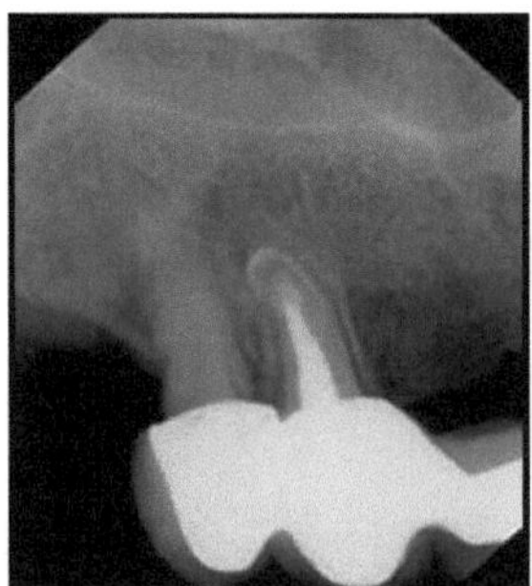

Figure 52: Radiological check at 3 weeks postoperatively. [21]

■ Four years postoperatively: Favorable clinical and radiological outcome (Figures 53 and 54)

Periapical radiography at 4 years showed good apical healing and signs of bone regeneration.

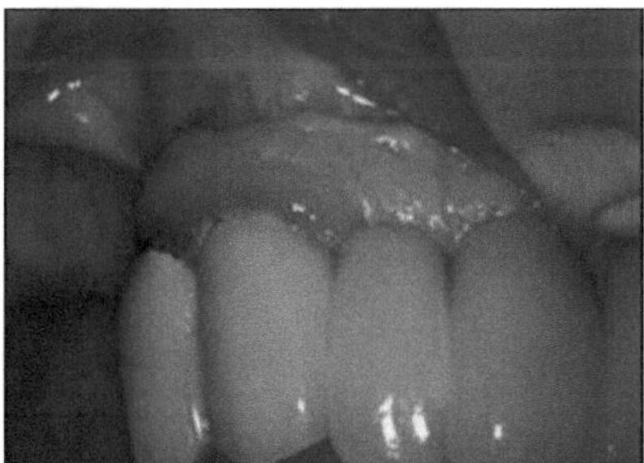

Figure 53: Clinical check-up at 4 years postoperatively. [21]

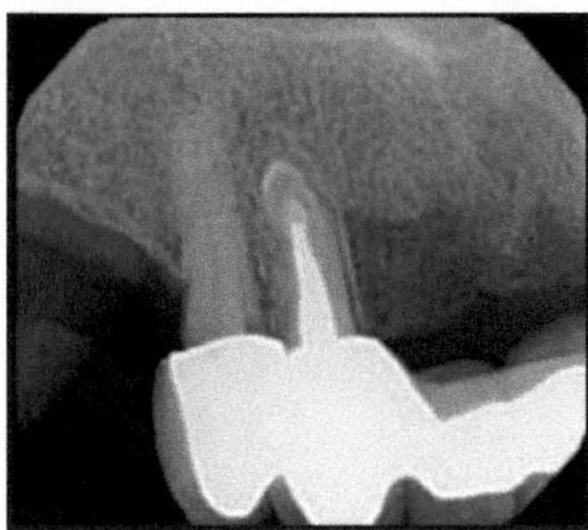

Figure 54: Periapical radiograph at 4 years postoperatively. [21]

Comparison of Er:YAG and Er,Cr:YSÇÇ lasers in the literature

Although the two laser systems, Er: YAG and Er, Cr: YSGG, are very similar in terms of design and basic characteristics, the difference in their wavelength, output energy and pulse duration range has a significant influence on the quality and duration of laser treatment. [27]

These parameters will therefore be a reference for choosing the most appropriate Erbium laser for our dental practice.

1. Tissue penetration depth and cutting efficiency

The penetration depth of Erbium radiation into hard dental tissue is essentially related to its wavelength and the water content of the tissue.

The study by Diaci and Gaspirc in 2012, revealed that the wavelength of the Er: YAG laser (2940 nm) coincides with the water absorption peak (1200 mm-1) whereas that of the Er, Cr: YSGG laser (2780 nm) is three times lower (400 mm-1) [27] (Figure 55).

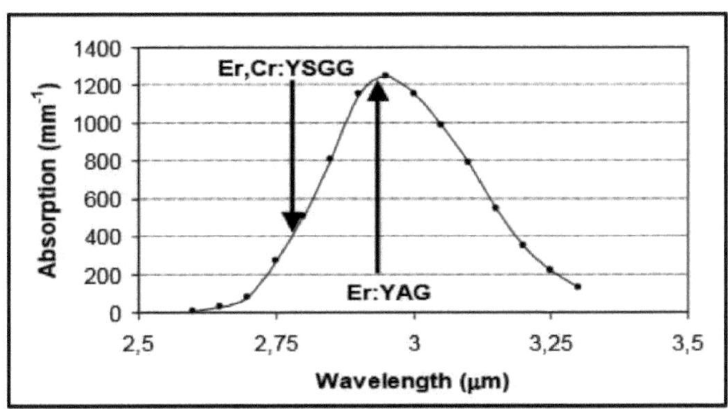

Figure 55: Absorption curve for water in the mid-infrared wavelength range.

Due to the different water content of hard dental tissues, the absorption coefficients of the Er:YAG laser were around 150 mm-1 in enamel and 200 mm-1 in dentin. The corresponding absorption coefficients for the Er, Cr: YSGG laser were three times lower [68].

This difference in absorption means that the wavelength of the Er:YAG laser penetrates around 7 micrometers into enamel and 5 micrometers into dentin. Whereas the Er, Cr: YSGG laser penetrates deeper, 21 micrometers into enamel and 15 micrometers into dentin, and therefore causes more thermal damage to tissue (Figure 56).

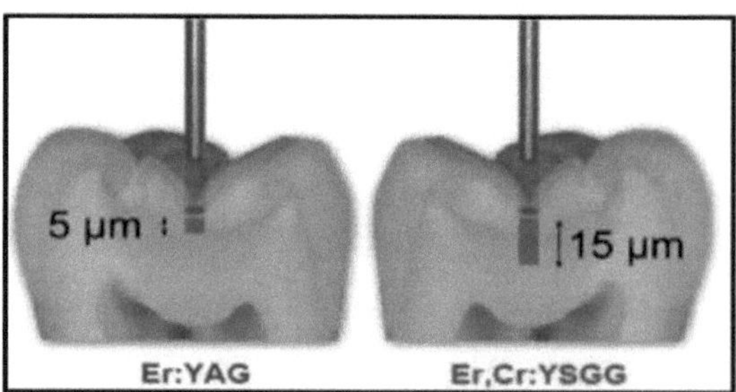

Figure 56: Penetration depths of Er: YAG and Er, Cr: YSGG lasers in dentin thickness. [1]

So, thanks to its higher absorption, the Er:YAG laser has a smaller penetration depth but more effective tissue ablation.

It therefore requires less energy and less time to ablate hard dental tissue compared with the Er, Cr: YSGG laser [27, 68].

In addition to wavelength, one of the key factors determining the efficacy and safety of laser ablation is the duration of the laser pulse. Indeed, if the required energy is delivered to the target tissue in a short time, it has little time to escape from the ablated tissue, thus increasing ablation efficiency. (Lukac et al in 2004)

Perhavec and Diaci in 2008 conducted an in vitro study to compare the ablation rate of hard dental tissue by Er: YAG and Er, Cr: YSGG lasers used at the same output energy (260 mJ) but different pulse durations [68].

The results of this study showed that the volume of dentin ablated per Er: YAG laser energy pulse (0.073 mm^3/J) was greater by a factor of 1.4 than that removed by the Er, Cr: YSGG laser (0.053 mm^3/J).

In enamel, the volume ablated per energy pulse of the Er: YAG laser (0.032mm^3/J) was a factor of 1.5 higher than that achieved by the Er, Cr: YSGG laser (0.021mm3/J).

This difference in ablation rate has been attributed to the fact that the Er:YAG laser offers the advantage of varying pulse durations, and can work at short pulses (up to 50μs).

In contrast, the Er, Cr: YSGG laser was limited to minimum pulse durations in excess of 400μs due to the long relaxation time of the Cr3+ ion.

The authors of this study concluded that, with similar settings for both laser systems, the Er:YAG laser offers superior performance in terms of ablation volumes.

2. Thermal damage caused

The greater the penetration depth of a laser, the more secondary thermal damage it causes.

In 2009, Perhavec et al conducted an in vitro study to compare residual heat deposition in teeth after tissue ablation with the Er: YAG laser (2490nm) and the Er, Cr: YSGG laser (2780 nm) [69].

In this study 3 types of Erbium laser were used with the same output energy (100 mJ) but different pulse modes:

- The Er: YAG laser (AT Fidelis, Fotona) with MSP "Medium Short Pulse" mode: pulse duration of 150μs.

- Er, Cr: YSGG laser in H mode (Waterlase, Biolase): pulse duration between 500 and 700 μs.
- The Er, Cr: YSGG laser in S mode (Waterlase, Biolase): pulse duration between 1200 and 1400 μs.

The study showed that the amount of unwanted residual heat remaining deposited in the tooth for the Er, Cr: YSGG laser was twice as great for the H mode and 3 times greater for the S mode than the heat deposited using the Er: YAG laser's MSP mode.

Thermal damage in the form of brownish spots was observed in the dentine of teeth irradiated with the Er, Cr: YSGG laser, despite the water spray used during treatment.

These authors also measured the maximum temperature increase in hard dental tissues (enamel and dentin) after irradiation with Erbium lasers.

They revealed that the temperature rise was more marked for the Er, Cr: YSGG laser (used in both H and S pulse modes) compared with the Er:

YAG laser (Figure 57).

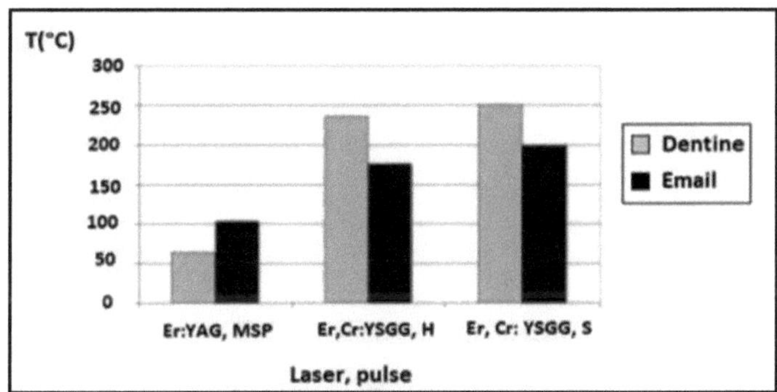

Figure 57: Temperature rise in dental tissue (enamel + dentine) as a function of laser pulse mode. [69]

Similarly, Diaci and Gaspirc in 2012 revealed that after Erbium laser irradiation without the use of water spray, the areas of thermal necrosis generated by the Er, Cr: YSGG laser were around three times greater than those caused by the Er: YAG laser [27].

The authors concluded that one of the main advantages of clinical use of the Er:YAG laser is its ability to remove both hard and soft dental tissue with minimal thermal damage.

3. Processing time

The greater the penetration depth of laser radiation, the greater the volume of irradiated tissue to be heated, and the slower the time required to reach ablation temperature.

Diaci and Gaspirc in 2012 showed that the Er, Cr: YSGG laser (2780nm), due to its greater penetration into hard dental tissue, requires around 3 times longer than the Er: YAG laser to heat the irradiated tissue volume to its ablation temperature [27].

As a result, tissue ablation started later with the Er, Cr: YSGG laser than with the Er: YAG laser.

This delay in the removal of dental tissue by the Er, Cr: YSGG laser was also attributed to the fact that some of the laser energy was dissipated in the surrounding tissue as the laser beam progressed deeper into the target tissue [28].

4. Type of pain felt

A study carried out by Claire Alamarguy in 2011 evaluated the type of pain experienced by the two lasers Er: YAG (2940 nm) and Er, Cr: YSGG (2780 nm) during dental treatment [2].

The results of this study showed that treatment with these two laser systems was generally painless for patients compared to conventional burr treatment.

Nevertheless, the pain generated, if any, was more tolerable with the Er: YAG laser than with the Er, Cr: YSGG laser (Figure 58).

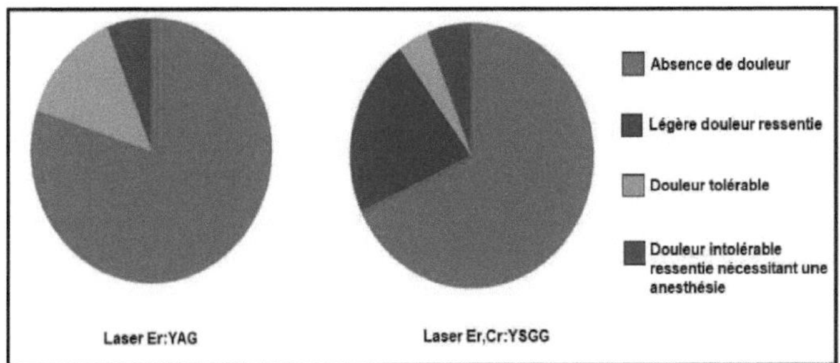

Figure 58: Representative diagrams of the pain experienced when using Er: YAG and Er, Cr: YSGG lasers. [2]

5. Conclusion

Despite the almost identical results of published studies, it seems that the Er:YAG laser is more recommended in our conservative dentistry and endodontics practice, since it combines the efficacy, safety, comfort and rapidity of LASER-assisted dental treatment.

Studies with a high level of scientific proof are still needed on this subject.

Conclusion

Conclusion

For modern, minimally invasive dentistry, Er: YAG (2940 nm) and Er, Cr: YSGG (2780 nm) lasers represent state-of-the-art technology for a wide range of clinical applications in conservative dentistry and endodontics.

Thanks to their versatility, these lasers are ideally suited to the treatment of both hard and soft dental tissue, with promising results.

In restorative dentistry, their effectiveness has been demonstrated in most clinical indications: precise and selective removal of carious lesions, etching of tooth surfaces for better adhesion of composite resin, and non-contact (vibration- and noise-free) treatment of tooth surfaces. These lasers have also made it possible to treat dentine sensitivity with significantly higher therapeutic success rates than conventional techniques.

In endodontics, Erbium lasers are used to prepare access cavities, find canal entrances and decontaminate the endodontic system by direct irradiation of canal walls and/or activation of irrigation solutions.

These lasers are also used to soften gutta-percha by photothermal effect and propel it through all main and accessory canals, optimizing the seal of the final root canal filling.

Added to this, Er: YAG and Er, Cr: YSGG lasers offer undeniable advantages in apical surgery: a single instrument for gingival incision, bone drilling, apex resection and decontamination of the surgical site, with excellent bone healing and pain-free, patient-acceptable postoperative follow-up.

However, despite their virtues, the literature has shown that Erbium lasers do not yet cover all clinical indications in OCE, and must often be combined with other LASER devices (such as the Diode laser for caries diagnosis). In addition, the slow clinical application time and high cost of these lasers still limit their use to dental practices.

A major challenge for researchers in the future is to develop less expensive, more versatile and more ergonomic devices, and why not the development of a Laser device integrating the qualities of several wavelengths, enabling it to broaden the scope of its clinical applications in dentistry.

References

References

1. Abdulsamee N.

Erbium Family Laser: Silent Revolution in Dentistry. Review.

EC Dental Science 2017; 13: 168-90.

2. Alamarguy C.

Lasers and their uses in conservative dentistry.

[Thesis]. Université Nancy Poincare-Nancy1, 2011.

3. Al-Batayneh OB, Seow WK, Walsh LJ.

Assessment of Er:YAG Laser for CavityPreparation in Primary and Permanent Teeth: A Scanning Electron Microscopy and Thermographic Study.

Pediatr Dent 2014; 36 (3): 90-4.

4. Amasyali M, Sabuncuoglu FA, Ersahan S, Oktay EA.

Comparison of the Effects of Various Methods Used to Remove Adhesive from Tooth Surfaces on Surface Roughness and Temperature Changes in the Pulp Chamber.

Turk J Orthod2019; 32(3):132-8.

5. Angiero F, Benedicenti S, Signore A, Parker S, Crippa R.

Apicoectomies with the erbium laser: acomplementary technique for retrograde endodontic treatment.

PhotomedLaser Surg 2011; 29(12): 845-9.

6. Aranha ACC, by Paulo Eduardo C.

Effects of Er: YAG and Er, Cr: YSGG lasers on dentine hypersensitivity. Shortterm clinical evaluation.

Lasers MedSci 2012; 27(4): 813-8.

7. **Aricioglu B, Arslan I, Duymus ZY. Çelik D.**

Comparison of calcium hydroxide removal efficacy of different

irrigation systems and photon-induced photoacustic streaming

technique.

JDental Lasers 2018; 12(1): 31.

8. **Arslan H, Akcay M, Capar ID, Saygili G, Gok T, Erats H.**

An in vitro comparison of irrigation using photon-initiated

photoacoustic streaming, ultrasonic, sonic and needle techniques in

removing calcium hydroxide.

Int Endod J 2015; 48(3): 246-51.

9. **Ayranci LB, Koseoglu M.**

The evaluation of the effects of different irrigating solutions and laser

systems on adhesion of resin-based root canal sealers.

PhotomedLaser Surg 2014; 32(3): 152-9.

10. **Baraba A, Kqiku L, Gabric D, Verzak Z, Hanscho K, Miletic I.**

Efficacy of removal of cariogenic bacteria and carious dentin by

ablation using different modes of Er: YAGlasers.

Braz JMedBiol Res 2018; 51(3) :6872.

11. **Baraba A, Perhavec T, Chieffi N, Ferrari M, Anic I, Miletic I.**

Ablative potential of four different pulses of Er: YAG lasers and low-

speed handpiece.

PhotomedLaser Surg 2012; 30(6): 301-7.

12. **Bagaran EG, Ayna E, Basaran G, Beydemir K.**

Influence of different power outputs of erbium, chromium: yttrium-

scandiumgallium-garnet laser and acid etching on shear bonds trengths of a dual-cure resin cement to enamel.

Lasers MedSci 2011; 26(1):13-9.

13. Bertrand MF, Rocca JP.

Er:YAG laser and restorative dentistry.

EMC-Stomatologie2005; 1 :104-115.

14. Blanken J, De Moor RJ, Meire M, Verdaasdonk R.

Laser induced explosive vapor and cavitation resulting in effective

irrigation of the root canal. Part 1 :avisualization study.

Lasers Surg Med 2009; 41(7) :514-9.

15. Bodrumlu E, Keskiner I, Sumer M, Sumer AP, Telcioglu NT.

Temperature variation during apicectomy with Er:YAG laser.

PhotomedLaser Surg 2012; 30(8): 425-8.

16. Shah S.

The erbium laser in restorative-endodontic dentistry. [Thesis].

Lille 2 University of Law and Health: Faculty of Dental Surgery;

2018.

17. Cartwright RB.

Dentinal hypersensitivity: a narrative review Community.

Dental Health 2014; 31: 1-6.

18. Ceballos-Jiménez AY, Rodríguez-Vilchis LE, Contreras-Bulnes R.

Chemical Changes of Enamel Produced by Sodium Fluoride,

Hydroxyapatite, Er:YAG Laser, and Combined Treatments.

Journal of Spectroscopy 2018; 7.

19. Cengiz E, Yilmaz HG.

Efficacy of Erbium, Chromium-doped: Yttrium, Scandium, Gallium, and Garnet Laser Irradiation Combined with Resin-based Tricalcium Silicate and Calcium Hydroxide on Direct Pulp Capping: A Randomized Clinical Trial.

JEndod 2016; 42(3):351-5.

20. Chen ML, Ding JF, He YJ, Chen Y, Jiang Q.

Effect of pretreatment on Er: YAG laser-irradiated dentin.

Lasers MedSci 2015; 30(2):753-9.

21. Chen WH.

Apicoectomy Performed Using the Er, Cr: YSGG Laser System: A Case Report. 2020

22. Cheng X, Xiang D, He W, Qiu J, Han B, Yu Q, Tian Y.

Bactericidal effect of Er: YAG laser-activated sodium hypochlorite irrigation against biofilms of Enterococcus faecalis isolate from canal of root-filled teeth with periapical lesions. *PhotomedLaser Surg 2017; 35 (7): 386-92.*

23. David CM, Gupta P.

Lasers in Dentistry: A Review.

Int JAdv Health Sci2015 ;2 :7-13.

24. De Oliveira RM, de Souza VM, Esteves CM, Lima-Arsati YB, Cassoni A, Rodrigues JA et al.

Er, Cr:YSGG Laser Energy Delivery: Pulse and Power Effects on Enamel Surface and Erosive Resistance.

PhotomedLaser Surg 2017; 35(11):639-46.

25. Deng Y, Zhu X, Zheng D, Yan P, Jiang H.

Laser use in direct pulp capping: A meta-analysis.

J Am Dent Assoc 2016; 147(12): 935-42.

26. Deponte S.

The erbium laser in endodontics.

AO News 2018.

27. Diaci J, Gaspirc, B.

Comparison of Er: YAG and Er, Cr : YSGG lasers used in dentistry.

JLaser healthAcad 2012; 1(1): 1-13.

28. Diaci J.

Laser profilometry for the characterization of craters produced in hard dental tissues by Er: YAG and Er, Cr : YSGG lasers.

JLaser HealthAcademy 2008; 2: 15-20.

29. Díaz-Monroy JM, Contreras-Bulnes R, Olea-Mejía OF.

Chemical changes associated with increased acid resistance of Er:YAG laser irradiated enamel.

The Scientific World Journal 2014 : 1-6.

30. Divito E, Crippa R, Laria G.

Lasers in endodontics.

Laser 2012; 2: 18-26.

31. Geraldo-Martins VR, Penazzo Lepri C, Palma-Dibb RG.

Influence of Er, Cr: YSGG laser irradiation on enamel caries prevention.

Lasers Med Sci 2013; 28: 33-9.

32. Golob BS, Olivi G, Vrabec M, El Feghali R, Parker S, Benedicenti S.

Efficacy of Photon-induced Photoacoustic Streaming in the Reduction of Enterococcus faecalis within the Root Canal: Different Settings and Different Sodium Hypochlorite Concentrations.

JEndod 2017; 43(10): 1730-5.

33. Gorduysus MO, Al-Rubai H, Salman B, Al Saady D, Al-Dagistani H, Muftuoglu S.

Using erbium-doped yttrium aluminumgarnet laser irradiation in different energy output levels versus ultrasonic in removal of root canal filling materials in endodontic retreatment.

Eur JDent 2017; 11(3) :281-6.

34. Harashima T, Kinoshita JI, Kimura Y, Brugnera A, Zanin F, Pecora JD et al.

Morphological Comparative Study on Ablation of Dental Hard

Tissues at Cavity Preparation by Er:YAG and Er, Cr: YSGG Lasers.

Photomed Laser Surg 2005; 23: 52-5.

35. Hossain M, Nakamura Y, Yamada Y, Suzuki N, Murakami Y, Matsumoto K.

Analysis of Surface Roughness of Enamel and DentinafterEr, Cr:

YSGG Laser Irradiation.

J Clin Laser MedSurg 2001; 19(6): 297-303.

36. Inamoto K, Horiba N, Senda S et al.

Possibility of root canal preparation by Er:YAG laser.

Oral Surg Oral Med Oral Pathol Oral RadiolEndod.2009 ; 107(1) : e47-55.

37. Jaramillo DE.

Irrigation of root canal system by laser activation (LAI): PIPS Photon-Induced Photoacoustic Streaming.

Endodontic Irrigation.Springer 2015.227-235.

38. **Kallis A.**

Case Report: The Use of 2940 nm Er: YAG Laser in Cavity Preparation.

JLaser Health Academy 2014; 1: 1855-1913.

39. **Keles A, Arslan H, Kamalak A, Akacay M, Sousa-Neto MD, Versiani MA.**

Removal of filling materials fromoval-shaped canals using laser irradiation: a micro-computed tomographic study.

JEndod2015; 41(2): 219-24.

40. **Khatavkar R, Hegde V.**

Surface analysis of Erbium:YAG laser etching compared with acid etching.

Laser 2012; 2:42-5.

41. **Kihara T, Matsumoto H. Yoshimine Y.**

Evaluation of the efficacy of Er: YAG laser-activated irrigation in a simulated accessory canal.

JDental Lasers 2019; 13(2): 34.

42. **Kilinc E, Roshkind DM, Antonson SA, Antonson DE, Hardigan PC, Siegel SC et al.**

Thermal safety of Er: YAG and Er,Cr : YSGG lasers in hard tissue removal.

PhotomedLaser Surg 2009;27(4): 565-70.

43. **Kokuzawa C, Ebihara A, Watanabe S et al.**

Shaping of the root canal using Er:YAG laser irradiation.

PhotomedLaser Surg. 2012; 30(7):367-73.

44. **Kolnick J.**

The clinical use of the Er, Cr: YSGG laser in endodontic therapy.

Roots 2011; 2:14-8.

45. **Komabayashi T, Ebihara A, Aoki A.**

The use of lasers for direct pulp capping.

J Oral Sci 2015; 57(4): 277-86.

46. **Kumar P, Goswami M, Dhillon JK, Rehman F, Thakkar D, Bharti K.**

Comparative evaluation of microhardness and morphology of permanent toothenamel surface after laser irradiation and fluoride treatment-An in vitro study.

Laser Ther 2016 ;25(3) :201-8.

47. **Laky M, Volmer M, Arslan M, Agis H, Moritz A, Cvikl B.**

Efficacy and Safety of Photon Induced Photoacoustic Streaming for Removal of Calcium Hydroxide in Endodontic Treatment.

BiomedRes Int 2018 ; 2018: 2845705.

48. **Laria G, Crippa R, Olivi G.**

Use of Er, Cr: YSGG and Er:YAG lasers in restorative dentistry.

Laser 2011; 1: 31-4.

49. **Li T, Zhang X, Shi H, Ma Z, Lv B, Xie M.**

Er: YAG laser application in caries removal and cavity preparation in children: a meta-analysis.

Lasers MedSci 2019; 34(2): 273-80.

50. **Lietzau M, Smeets R, Hanken H, Heiland M, Apel C.**

Apicoectomy using Er:YAG laser in association with microscope: a comparative retrospective investigation.

PhotomedLaser Surg 2013; 31(3):110-5.

51. Lima DM, Tonetto MR, de Mendonça AAM, Elossais AA, Saad JRC, de Andrade MF et al.

Human dental enamel and dentin structural effects after Er: YAG laser irradiation.

J Contemp Dent Pract 2014; 15(3): 283-7.

52. Lin S, Liu Q, Peng Q.

The ablation threshold of Er: YAG laser and Er, Cr: YSGG laser in dental dentin.

SciResearchEssays 2010; 5(16):2128-35.

53. Liu Y, Hsu CY, Teo CM, Teoh SH.

Potential mechanism for the laser-fluoride effect on enamel demineralization.

JDent Res 2013; 92(1): 71-5.

54. Liu Y, Hsu CY, Teo CM, Teoh SH.

SubablativeEr: YAG laser effect on enamel demineralization.

Caries Res 2013; 47(1): 63-8.

55. Lopes RM, Trevelin LT, da Cunha SRB, de Oliviera RF, Salgado DMR, de Freitas PM et al.

Dental Adhesion to Erbium-Lased Tooth Structure: A Review of the Literature.

PhotomedLaser Surg 2015; 33(8):393-403.

56. Matos AB, De Azevedo CS, Da Ana PA.

Laser technology for caries removal.

Contemporary Approach to Dental Caries 2012; 1: 292-312.

57. **Matsumoto H, Yoshimine Y, Akamine A.**

Visualization of irrigant flow and cavitation induced by Er: YAG laser within a root canal model.

JEndod2010; 37(6): 839-43.

58. **Mazeki K, Kimura Y, Yokoyama K, Matsumoto K.**

Preparation of root canal orifices by Er:YAG laser irradiation: in vitro and clinical observations.

J Clin Laser MedSurg 2003;21(2) :85-91.

59. **Meire MA, Havelaerts S, De Moor RJ.**

Influence of lasing parameters on the cleaning efficacy of laser-activated irrigation with pulsed erbium lasers.

Lasers MedSci 2016; 31(4) :653-8.

60. **Minas NH, Meister J, Franzen R, Gutknecht N, Lampert F, Mir M.**

In vitro preliminary study to evaluate the capability of Er, Cr: YSGG laser in posterior teeth root-canal preparation with step-back technique.

Lasers Med Sci 2009; 24(1): 7-12.

61. **Molaasadollah F, Asnaashari M, Abbas FM, Jafary M.**

In vitro comparison of fluoride gel alone and in combination with Er, Cr: YSGG laser on reducing white spot lesions in primary teeth.

JLasers Med Sci Fall 2017; 8(4): 160-5.

62. **Moosavi H, Ghorbanzadeh S, Ahrani F.**

Structural and Morpholigical Changes in Human Dentin after Ablative and SubablativeEr: YAG Laser Irradiation.

JLasers MedSci 2016; 7(2):86-91.

63. **Negi S, Adhikari HD, Mazumder D, Deirimika L, Bhardwaj S.**

Comparative evaluation of microleakage after root-end resection by erbium, chromium: Yttrium-scandium-gallium-garnet (Er, Cr: YSGG) laser and carbide bur with or without placement of mineral trioxide aggregate: An in vitro study. *J Conserv Dent 2019; 22(4): 391.*

64. **Olivi G, De Moor R, DiVito E.**

Lasers in endodontics: scientific back ground and clinical applications.

Springer; 2016.

65. **Olivi G, DiVito E, Peters O, Kaitsas V, Angiero F, Signore A et al.**

Disinfection efficacy of photon-induced photoacoustic streaming on root canals infected with Enterococcus faecalis: an ex vivo study. *JAm Dent Assoc 2014; 145(8): 843-8.*

66. **Ozkocak I, Sonat B.**

Evaluation of Effects on the Adhesion of Various Root Canal Sealers after Er: YAG Laser and Irrigants Are Used on the Dentin Surface. *JEndod2015; 41(8): 1331-6.*

67. **Ozlem K, Esad GM, Ayse A, Aslihan U.**

Efficiency of Lasers and a Desensitizer Agent on Dentin Hypersensitivity Treatment: A Clinical Study. *Niger J Clin Pract 2018; 21(2): 225-30.*

68. **Perhavec T, Diaci J.**

Comparison of Er:Yag and Er, Cr: YSGG dental lasers. *J Oral Laser App 2008; 8: 87-94.*

69. Perhavec T, Lukac M, Diaci J, Marincek M.

Heat deposition of erbium lasers in hard dental tissues.

J Oral Laser App 2009; 9(4): 205-12.

70. Poli R, Parker S.

Achieving Dental Analgesia with the Erbium Chromium Yttrium Scandium Gallium Garnet Laser (2780 nm): A Protocol for Painless Conservative Treatment.

Photomed Laser Surg 2015; 33(7): 364-71.

71. Poli R.

Laser-Assisted Restorative Dentistry (Hard Tissue: Carious Lesion Removal and Tooth Preparation).

Lasers in Dentistry-Current Concepts 2017; 8: 163-89.

72. Ramalho KM, Hsu CYS, de Freitas PM, Aranha ACC, Esteves-Oliveira M, Rocha RG.

Erbium Lasers for the Prevention of Enamel and Dentin Demineralization: A Literature Review.

Photomed Laser Surg 2015; 33(66): 301-19.

73. Raucci-Neto W, Dos Santos CR, de Lima FA, Pécora JD, Bachmann L, Palma-Dibb RG.

Thermal effects and morphological aspects of varying Er: YAG laser energy on demineralized dentin removal: an in vitro study.

Lasers Med Sci 2015; 30(4):1231-6.

74. Rey G, Girard J, Para A, Lamouret P, Missika P.

Use of lasers in endodontics.

Rueil-Malmaison: Edition CdP; 2014. 162 p

75. **Roper M J, White JM, Goodis HE.**

Two-dimensional changes and surface characteristics from an erbium laser used for root canal preparation.

Lasers Surg Med2010; 42(5): 379-83.

76. **Roszkiewicz P.**

Laser-assisted direct pulp capping.

Laser 2017; 3:16-8.

77. **Sahar-Helft S, Sarp ASK, Stabholtz A, Gutkin V, Redenski I, Steinberg D.**

Comparison of positive-pressure, passive ultrasonic, and laser-activated irrigations on smear-layer removal from the root canal surface.

PhotomedLaser Surg 2015; 33(3):129-35.

78. **Sahar-Helft S. Stabholtz A.**

Rermoving smear layer during endodontic treatment by different techniques-A in vitro study. A clinical case-Endodontic treatment with Er: YAG Laser.

Stomatol Edu J2016; 3:162-7.

79. **Santos CR, Tonetto M, Presoto CD.**

Application of Er:YAG and Er, Cr:YSGG Lasers in Cavity Preparation for Dental Tissues: A Literature Review.

World JDent 2012; 3(4): 340-3.

80. **Sarmadi R, Andersson EV, Lingstrom P, Gabre P.**

A Randomized Controlled Trial Comparing Er:YAG Laser and Rotary Bur in the Excavation of Caries - Patients' Experiences and the Quality of Composite Restoration.

Open Dent J 2018; 12: 443-54.

81. Silva AC, Melo P, Ferreira JC, Oliveira T, Gutknecht N.

Adhesion in Dentin Prepared with Er, Cr: YSGG Laser: Systematic Review.

Contemp Clin Dent 2019; 10(1): 129-34.

82. Strakas D, Gutknecht N.

Erbium lasers in operative dentistry - a literature review.

Lasers Dental Sci 2018; 2: 125-36.

83. Tachinami H, Katsuumi I.

Removal of root canal filling materials using Er: YAG laser irradiation.

Dent Mater J2010; 29(3): 246-52.

84. Tao S, Li L, Yuan H, Tao S, Cheng Y, He L et al.

Erbium laser technology Vs traditional drilling for caries removal: A systematic review with meta-analysis.

J Evid Based Dent Pract 2017; 17: 324-34.

85. Tsanova ST, Tomov GT.

Morphological changes in hard dental tissues prepared by Er:YAGLaser (LiteTouch, Syneron), Carisolv and rotary instruments. A scanning electron microscopy evaluation.

Folia Medica 2010; 52(3): 46-55.

86. van As G.

Erbium lasers in dentistry.

Dental Clinics 2004; 48 (4): 1017-1059.

87. Wang X, Cheng X, Liu B, Liu X, Yu Q, He W.

Effect of Laser-Activated Irrigations on Smear Layer Removal from the Root Canal Wall. *PhotomedLaser Surg 2017; 35(12): 688-94.*

88. Wang X, Cheng X, Liu X, Wang Z, Wang J, Guo C et al.

Bactericidal effect of various laser irradiation systems on enterococcus faecalis biofilms in dentinal tubules: A confocal laser scanning microscopy study.

PhotomedLaser Surg 2018; 36(9): 472-9.

89. Yassaei S, Aghili H, Joshan N.

Effects of removing adhesive from tooth surfaces by Er: YAG laser and a composite bur on enamel surface roughness and pulp chamber temperature.

Dent Research J 2015; 12(3): 254-9.

90. Yilmaz HG, Bayindir H.

Clinical and scanning electron microscopy evaluation of the Er, Cr: YSGG laser therapy for treating dentine hypersensitivity: short-term, randomised, controlled study.

J Oral Rehabil 2014; 41(5): 392-8.

91. Zhao XY, Wang S, Zhang CF.

Root resection by Er: YAG laser: a scanning electron microscope study.

West China JStomatol 2010; 28(5): 526-8.

92. Zhegova GG, Rashkova MR.

Er-YAG laser and dental caries treatment of permanent teeth in childhood.

JIMAB 2015; 21:699-704.

Internet references

93. Gaultier F, Navarro G.

Lasers in dentistry.

[Online]. 2013.[Accessed October 20, 2020]. Available from:

https://www.lefildentaire.com/ articles/practice/au-fil-des-

conferences/les-lasers- en-odontologie/

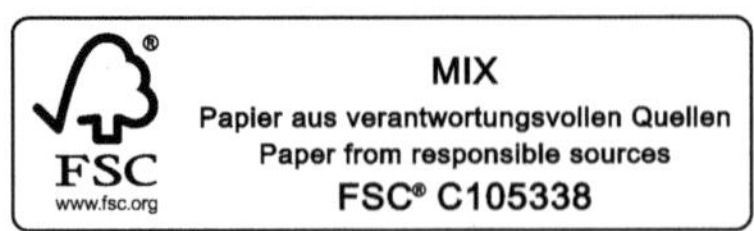

Printed by Books on Demand GmbH, Norderstedt / Germany